AF385717

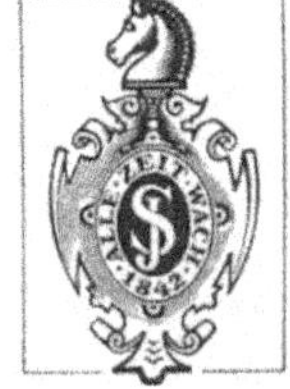

Surgery in Solitary Kidney and Corrections of Urinary Transport Disturbances

Volume Editors

L. Spitz, London
P. Wurnig, Vienna
Th. A. Angerpointner, Munich

With 136 Figures and 34 Tables

Springer-Verlag
Berlin Heidelberg New York
London Paris Tokyo

Professor Lewis Spitz, PhD, FRCS
Nuffield Professor of Pediatric Surgery, Institute of Child Health
30 Guilford Street, London WC1N 1EH, United Kingdom, and
Consultant Pediatric Surgeon, Hospital for Sick Children
Great Ormond Street, London, WC1N 3JH, United Kingdom

Primarius Professor Dr. Peter Wurnig
Chirurgische Abteilung des Mautner Markhof'schen Kinderspitals
der Stadt Wien, Baumgasse 75, 1030 Vienna, Austria

Priv.-Doz. Dr. Thomas A. Angerpointner
Kinderchirurgische Klinik im Dr. von Haunerschen Kinderspital
Lindwurmstraße 4, 8000 Munich 2, Federal Republic of Germany

Volumes 1–17 of this series were published
by Urban & Schwarzenberg, Baltimore–Munich

ISBN-13:978-3-642-74243-9   e-ISBN-13:978-3-642-74241-5
DOI: 10.1007/978-3-642-74241-5

Library of Congress Cataloging-in-Publication Data
Surgery in solitary kidney and corrections of urinary transport disturbances /
volume editors, L. Spitz, P. Wurnig, Th. A. Angerpointner.
p.   cm. − (Progress in pediatric surgery; v. 23)
Includes bibliographies and index.
ISBN-13:978-3-642-74243-9 (U.S.)
1. Genito-urinary organs − Surgery. 2. Children − Surgery. 3. Pediatric urology.
I. Spitz, Lewis. II. Wurnig, Peter. III. Angerpointner, Thomas.
[DNLM: 1. Genitalia − surgery. 2. Kidney − surgery. 3. Surgery, Plastic − in infancy & child-
hood. 4. Urinary Diversion − in infancy & childhood.   W1 PR677KA v. 23 / WJ 368 S961]
RD137.A1P7   vol. 23   [RD571]   617'.98 s − dc19   [617'.46]
DNLM/DLC   88-35477

2123/3145-543210   Printed on acid-free paper

Table of Contents

List of Editors

Angerpointner, T. A., Priv.-Doz. Dr., Kinderchirurgische Klinik im Dr. von Haunerschen Kinderspital der Universität München, Lindwurmstraße 4, D-8000 München 2

Gauderer, Michael, W. L., MD, University Pediatric Surgical Associates, 2101 Adelbert Road, Cleveland, OH 44106, USA

Hecker, W. Ch., Prof. Dr., Kinderchirurgische Klinik im Dr. von Haunerschen Kinderspital der Universität München, Lindwurmstraße 4, D-8000 München 2

Prévot, J., Prof., Clinique Chirurgical Pédiatrique, Hôpital d'Enfants de Nancy, F-54511 Vandœvre Cedex

Rickham, P. P., Prof. Dr. MD, MS, FRCS, FRCSI, FRACS, DCH, FAAP, Universitätskinderklinik, Chirurgische Abteilung, Steinwiesstraße 75, CH-8032 Zürich

Spitz, L., Prof., PhD, FRCS, Nuffield Professor of Pediatric Surgery, Institute of Child Health, University of London, Hospital for Sick Children, Great Ormond Street, 30 Guilford Street, GB-London WC1N 1EH

Stauffer, U. G., Prof. Dr., Universitätskinderklinik, Kinderchirurgische Abteilung, Steinwiesstraße 75, CH-8032 Zürich

Wurnig, P., Prof. Dr., Kinderchirurgische Abteilung des Mautner Markhof'schen Kinderspitals, Baumgasse 75, A-1030 Wien

List of Contributors

Part I

Surgery in Solitary Kidney

Value of Ultrasound in the Treatment
of Solitary Kidneys in Infancy and Childhood

H.-J. Beyer[1], V. Hofmann[2], and D. Brettschneider[2]

Summary

Every second patient with a solitary kidney suffers from renal disease. This accumulation of renal diseases of varying origin makes special care for these children necessary.

The quality of diagnostic methods is decisive for the choice of therapy. The advantages of primary ultrasound diagnosis and sonographical function tests are described. Sonographical differentiation of disturbances of the urinary transport is possible by means of forced-diuresis ultrasonography, whereas a vesico-ureteral reflux can be detected by means of voiding sonocystography.

The value of ultrasound for primary diagnosis, assessment of therapeutic course and postoperative long-term follow-up is discussed.

Zusammenfassung

Jeder zweite Patient mit einer Einzelniere ist nierenkrank. Die Häufung von Erkrankungen unterschiedlicher Genese ist Ursache der besonderen Sorge um diese Kinder.

Die Qualität der diagnostischen Methoden ist entscheidend bei der Wahl der Therapie. Es werden die Vorzüge der sonographischen Primärdiagnostik und der sonographischen Funktionsdiagnostik dargestellt. Die sonographische Differenzierung von Harntransportstörungen der Einzelniere ist mit Hilfe der forcierten Diuresesonographie möglich, während der vesicoureterale Reflux mit Hilfe der Miktions-Sonocystographie erfaßt werden kann.

Der Stellenwert der Sonographie bei der Primärdiagnostik, der Verlaufskontrolle und in der postoperativen Langzeitbeurteilung werden diskutiert.

Résumé

Un patient sur deux, avec un seul rein, est néphropathique. Ces enfants qui présentent le plus souvent un cumul d'affections d'étiologie diverse doivent évidemment faire l'objet d'une attention toute particulière.

[1] Ruhruniversität Bochum, Kinderchirurgische Klinik, Widumer Str. 8, 4690 Herne, FRG
[2] St. Barbara Hospital, Pediatric Surgery, Barbarastr. 3–5, 4020 Halle, German Democratic Republic

Progress in Pediatric Surgery, Vol. 23
Ed. by L. Spitz et al.
© Springer-Verlag Berlin Heidelberg 1989

La fiabilité des méthodes diagnostiques est d'une importance capitale pour le choix de la démarche thérapeutique à suivre. Les auteurs font état des avantages du diagnostique primaire et du diagnostique fonctionnel par échographie. L'échographie permet l'étude des affections des voies urinaires entravant le transport de l'urine dans le cas d'un rein unique par diurèse forcée et le reflux vésico-urétéral peut être mis en évidence par la cystosonographie durant la miction.

Les auteurs discutent de l'importance de l'échographie lors du diagnostic primaire, du contrôle de l'évolution et du pronostic à long terme après intervention chirurgicale.

Introduction

Congenital solitary kidney results from contralateral renal agenesis or aplasia, when only one kidney develops in the embryonic stage or the development of one kidney is disturbed, respectively. Acquired solitary kidney is caused by suspension of the function of one kidney (autonephrectomy) or by the removal of a non-functioning kidney (nephrectomy; Hofmann and Forth 1981).

Loss or agenesis of one kidney effects a compensatory enlargement of the residual kidney. Adaptation to increased performance is achieved either by hypertrophy (cell enlargement of the nephrons; Brod 1964; Rockstroh and Samtleben 1974) or by hyperplasia (cell neogenesis; Brod 1964; Rockstroh and Samtleben 1974; Stojkovio et al. 1972).

Evidently, the younger the patient, the greater is his or her capability for compensatory renal hypertrophy (Fida 1960; Stojkovio et al. 1972). It has also been shown that infections of the residual organ prevent compensatory hypertrophy (Fida 1960). There is agreement among various authors that the incidence of nephrological/urological diseases is much higher in patients with congenital solitary kidney or acquired residual kidney than in people with two kidneys (Fida 1960). Morbidity amounts to over 40% in children (Fukala et al. 1976) and to more than 50% in adults (Rockstroh 1967).

Thus, the solitary kidney, which itself can be considered a disease, must be given due regard. Diagnosis and the resulting treatment are of particular importance in disease of solitary kidneys. The indication for active surgical treatment or primary conservative therapy is determined by the quality of diagnostic methods. Two criteria are of decisive importance: (a) assessment of the morphology and (b) assessment of the function of the solitary kidney.

This is true not only for the primary diagnosis, but also particularly for follow-up after primary conservative or surgical therapy. As far as possible, diagnostic procedures should be non-invasive, low or non-irradiating and highly effective (Beyer 1985; Hofmann 1981).

Diagnostic Technique and Normal Findings

Primary Sonographical Examination

Considerable compensatory hypertrophy of the solitary kidney is often found during primary sonographical examination (Hofmann 1981); however this may not always be the case in a diseased solitary kidneys.

Above all, misinterpretations can occur with left-sided renal agenesis, since the spleen is frequently positioned in the renal bed. This organ, poor in echos and without a pelvic reflex band, can be misjudged as hydronephrosis. If no organ can be found in the normal position, a dystopic kidney (pelvic kidney, for instance) must always be searched for.

Intravenous pyelography must always be carried out for the final diagnosis of a solitary kidney and assessment of renal function.

Sonographically recognizable parameters are:

1. Position, size, delimitation of solitary kidney
2. Structure and width-thickness of renal parenchyma
3. Form and structure of the pelvic reflex band
4. Distal ureter, urinary bladder, width-thickness of bladder wall
5. Assessment of micturition free of residual urine

Systematic examinations of the urinary tract render a differentiation between anatomical norm variants and even slightly pathological changes possible. The following are sonographically recognizable pathological changes, for which treatment is usually surgical:

1. Disturbances of urinary transport (DUT)
   a) Subpelvic DUT
   b) Pre-/subvesical DUT
2. Reflux and/or reflux nephropathy
3. Nephrolithiasis
4. Cystic solitary kidney
5. Tumorous solitary kidney
6. Solitary kidney following trauma

The morphological changes of the kidney as seen sonographically will be described for each of these conditions and the corresponding assessment of function will be presented.

Disturbances of Urinary Transport

The parenchyma pelvis index (PPI) is derived from the ratio of parenchymal width to the pelvic reflex band. The normal value is 2:1. Morphological changes of the kidney and the urinary collecting system caused by DUT can also be disclosed sonographically. According to Williams (1974), DUT can be subdivided into two main groups: (a) proximal stenoses and (b) distal stenoses.

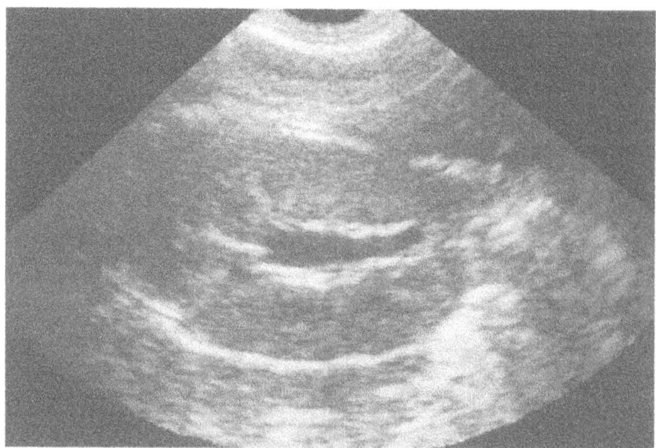

Fig. 1. Stage-I DUT: slight enlargement of the renal collecting system

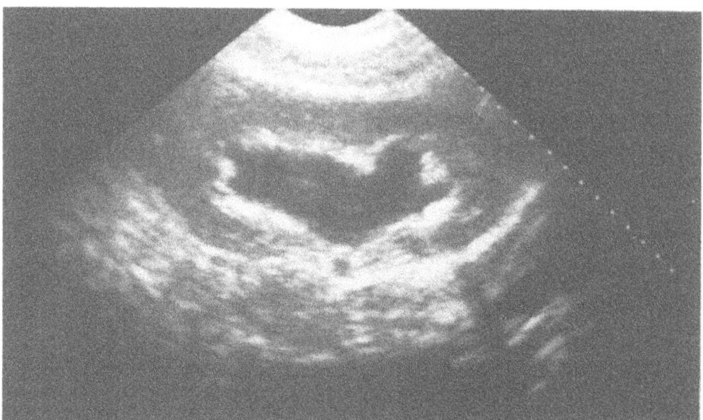

Fig. 2. Stage-II DUT: more pronounced enlargement of the renal collecting system

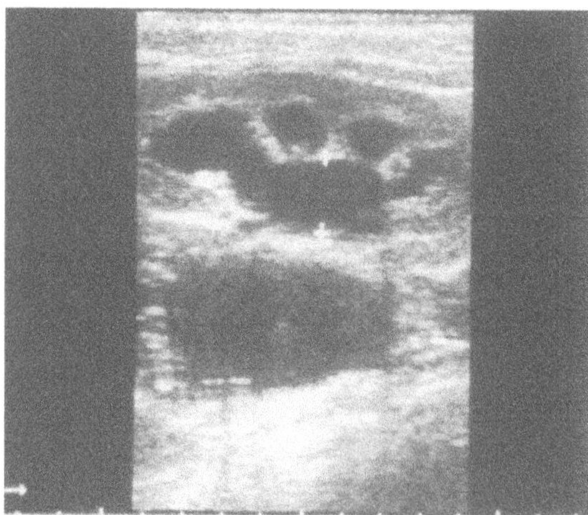

Fig. 3. Stage-III DUT: enlarged renal collecting system with fluid-filled renal calices

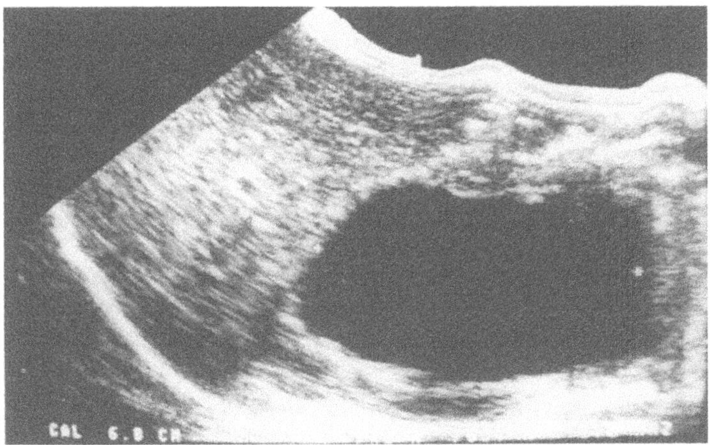

Fig. 4. Stage-IV DUT: massively enlarged pelvis with disappearance of renal calices

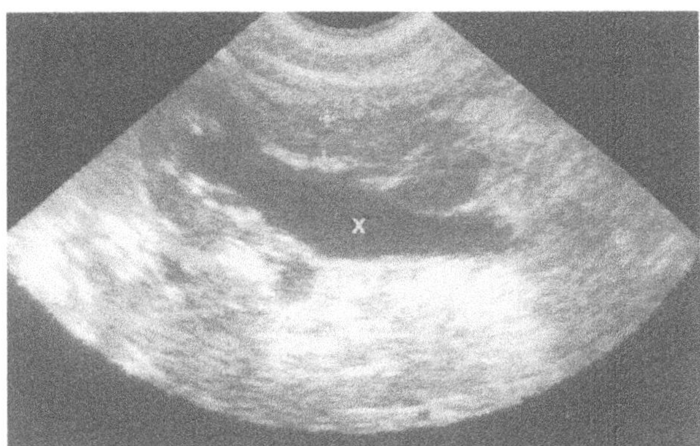

Fig. 5. Pronounced enlargement of the pelvis with proximally dilated ureter *(x)*

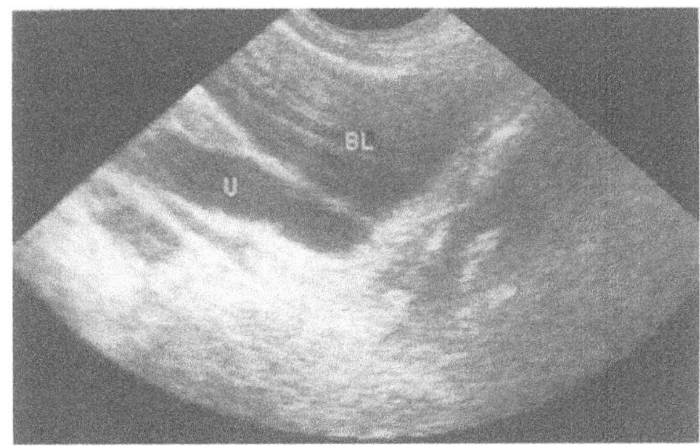

Fig. 6. Transverse section through the bladder *(BL)* with markedly dilated ureter *(U)*. (Figs. 5 and 6 correspond to a stage-III DUT in a distal ureteral stenosis)

Table 1. Classification of DUT in subpelvic stenosis

Stage of DUT	Normal finding	Stage I	Stage II	Stage III	Stage IV
Parenchymal width	Broad	Broad	Slightly diminished	Diminished	Parenchymal edge
Pelvis	Narrow	Slightly enlarged	Markedly enlarged	Grossly enlarged	Maximally enlarged
Parenchyma-pelvis index	2:1	2:1	1:2	1:3	1:4
Calices	Not visible	Not visible	Slightly enlarged	Markedly enlarged	Grossly enlarged
Ureter	–	–	–	–	–
Kidney, longitudinal section					
Kidney, transverse section					

Four stages of sonographically recognizable changes of the solitary kidney can be differentiated (Beyer 1984; Beyer and Hofmann 1985a):

- Stage I (slightly delayed urinary flow): the pelvis is not enlarged, and there is a small echo-free area in the pelvic reflex band; PPI 2:1 (Fig. 1)
- Stage II (delayed urinary flow): Enlargement of the pelvis. The broad reflex band is widely dispersed and encloses an echo-free area. The calices are not recognizable; the parenchyma is wide. PPI 1:1 (Fig. 2)
- Stage III (grossly delayed urinary flow): the pelvis is grossly enlarged; there is a small reflex band at the rim of a large echo-free area, and further small echo-free structures indicating caliceal enlargement. The parenchyma is diminished and seems to be, depending on the duration of DUT, more echogenic and less easily distinguishable from the surrounding tissue; PPI 1:2 (Fig. 3)
- Stage IV (maximally delayed urinary flow): the borders between the grossly enlarged pelvis and the massively dilated calices are no longer definable. There is no reflex band; only a small parenchymal edge can be seen at the rim of a large echo-free area. PPI 1:3 and more (Fig. 4)

Essentially, this classification is valid only for subpelvic ureteral stenoses (Table 1). The effect of distal stenoses on the urinary collecting system is relatively smaller: the ureter intercepts much of the volume and pressure so that the true extent of the stenosis can be determined only on examination of the distal ureter (Figs. 5 and 6; Table 2).

Table 2. Classification of DUT in distal obstruction

Stage of DUT	Normal finding	Stage I	Stage II	Stage III	Stage IV
Parenchymal width	Broad	Broad	Broad	Slightly diminished	Grossly diminished
Pelvis	Narrow	Slightly enlarged	Enlarged	Markedly enlarged	Maximally enlarged
Parenchyma-pelvis index	2:1	2:1	1:1	1:2	1:3
Calices	Not visible	Not visible	Not visible	Partly dilated	Grossly dilated
Ureter	Not visible	Narrow distally	Narrow distally and proximally	Distally and proximally marked	Distally and proximally wide
Kidney, longitudinal section					
Kidney, transverse section					
Bladder, longitudinal section					
Bladder, transverse section					

For the assessment of DUT it is essential to know whether the functional impairment of urinary flow is obstructive or non-obstructive. This important question can be answered by forced-diuresis ultrasound (FDU; Dinkel et al. 1982).

A picture of the kidney is made after the patient has consumed a normal breakfast (normal hydration) and the parameters parenchymal width, pelvic width and stage of DUT are assessed and photographically documented. Thereafter, the child is given 0.5 mg/kg furosemide, up to a maximal dose of 20 mg, and 20 ml/kg tea and repeated sonographical examinations are begun. Examinations are performed quarter-hourly during the first hour and then hourly until the initial values are reached. Those uropathies are assessed as non-obstructive DUT which allow a return of initial values after 3 h or sooner. Where an increase from stage II to stage IV lasts longer than 3 h, an obstructive uropathy requiring surgical treatment can be assumed. The same is true if the initial values correspond to a stage-III DUT. FDU is unnecessary in primary stage-IV DUT; however, the site of obstruction must be determined. Ultrasonography of the kidneys should always be performed

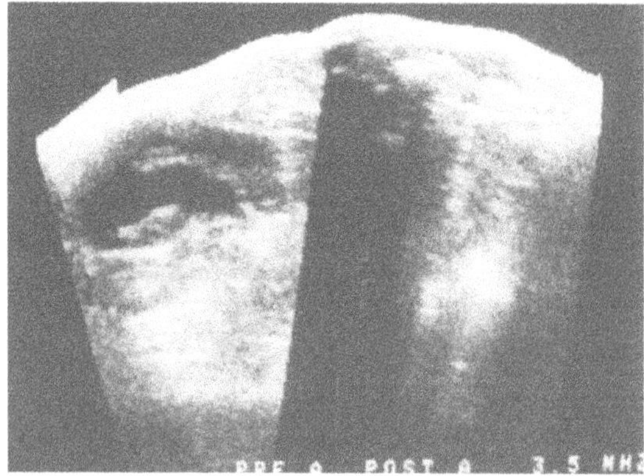

Fig. 7. Transverse section of a stage-II DUT − initial finding before forced diuresis

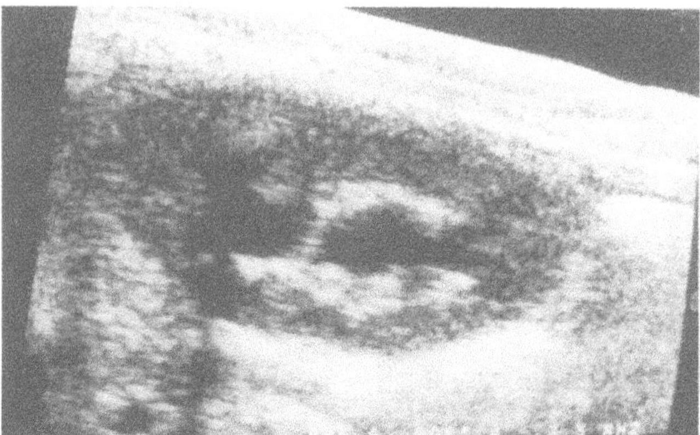

Fig. 8. Longitudinal section of a stage-II DUT-initial finding before forced diuresis

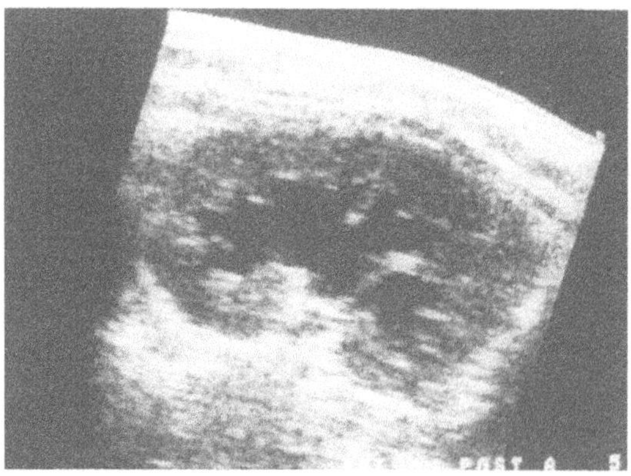

Fig. 9. Thirty minutes after the beginning of forced diuresis − stage-III DUT with caliceal enlargement

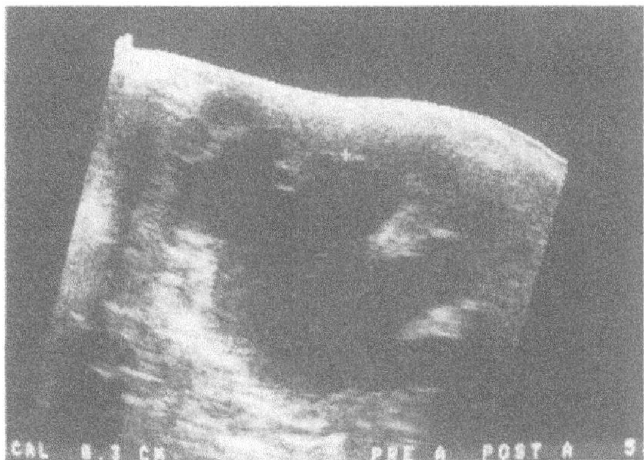

Fig. 10. Three hours later; a stage-III to -IV DUT is still present. (Figs. 7–10 correspond to an obstructive uropathy)

before and after voiding, since the distal ureter can be judged only when the bladder is full, but an objective assessment of the DUT stage is possible only when the bladder is empty. Results of examination in subpelvic and pre- and subvesical obstruction are very divergent. Whereas there is a very quick dilatation of the renal collecting system with subpelvic stenoses, distal stenoses primarily effect a dilatation of the ureter. The ureter is able to take up a relatively large volume of fluid before a change of the pre-existing DUT occurs (Figs. 7–10).

This sonographical functional test renders two essential statements possible: (a) differentiation between obstructive and non-obstructive uropathy, and (b) determination of the site of obstruction. An extended, but invasive, diagnostic method is ultrasound-guided puncture of the renal pelvis allowing antegrade pyelography and temporary urinary drainage.

We are of the opinion that the Whitaker test is no longer indicated, since further results cannot be expected.

Vesico-ureteral Reflux and Reflux Nephropathy

A dilatation of the intrarenal pelvis which normalizes quickly after micturition is a sign of vesico-ureteral reflux (VUR). VUR of long duration with recurrent urinary infections results in typical *reflux nephropathy:* the kidney is smaller than normal (limited compensatory hypertrophy); the parenchyma is more echogenic and poorly distinguishable from the surrounding tissue; there is a humpbacked renal contour.

For diagnosis and classification of VUR we perform voiding sonocystography (VSC; Beyer 1985; Beyer and Hofmann 1985b). Preparation and performance are the same as for conventional micturition cystourethrography (MCU). Following insertion of a Foley catheter and voiding of the bladder, the child is placed in a prone position. Renal parameters are measured and documented from the back. Thereafter, the bladder is filled with physiological salt solution; during filling, the kidney is continuously examined via longitudinal section. If there is a sonographi-

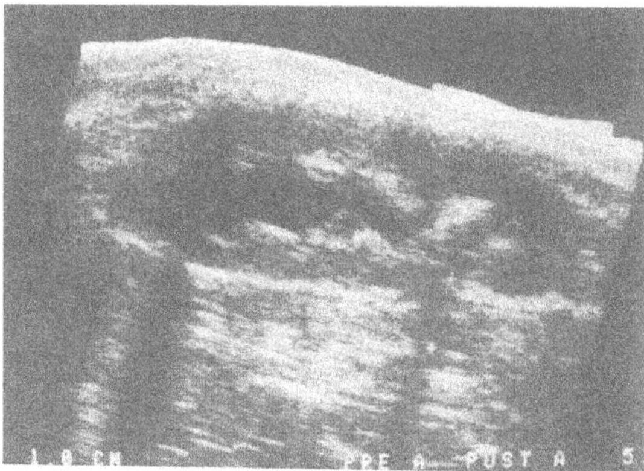

Fig. 11. Stage-II DUT in pelvic calculus. *+ +*, Echo-free area

cally recognizable dilatation of the renal collecting system during filling of the bladder, the child is brought into a supine position and the distal ureter is examined ventrally. In this functional test, it is essential to assess the pelvis and distal ureter when the bladder is empty, when it is full, and while it is being voided.

If there is already a dilatation of the renal collecting system during filling of the bladder, a low-pressure reflux can be assumed. If this is the case only after complete filling or during micturition, however, a high-pressure reflux must be present. Finally, it must be assessed whether micturition ensues free of residual urine. VSC allows the diagnosis of VUR combined with subvesical obstruction. The amount of bladder contents ascending to the pelvis determines the stage of VUR. All stage-II to -IV refluxes can be revealed by this method (Beyer 1985; Beyer and Hofmann 1985b). If the VSC shows evidence of a stage-II reflux or higher, an MCU is performed during the same session.

Nephrolithiasis

Diagnosis of nephrolithiasis can be made on the first attempt, if there is a calculus with a diameter of more than 3 mm in the renal pelvis. Calculi can effect a sonographically recognizable impairment of urinary flow (Fig. 11). Ureteral calculi, on the other hand, can mostly be seen only in the proximal or distal ureter. Besides the typical clinical picture, an obstructed pelvis or the ureter dilated proximal to the calculus are signs of ureteral calculi (Hofmann 1981).

Cystic Solitary Kidney

This very rare entity is characterized by solitary or multiple, round, echo-free and sharply defined areas within the parenchyma. It is difficult to decide whether there is a connection with the renal pelvis. In uncertain cases, ultrasound-guided puncture and filling of the "cystic" cavity can help to clarify whether a cyst is indeed present.

Solitary Kidney with Tumor

Various tumours of the kidney are known in childhood. A differentiation of the echo texture is possible by means of ultrasound. If the tumour is solid, neuroblastomas and Wilms' tumours can be distinguished since both neoplasms have a characteristic echo texture (Hofmann 1981).

Solitary Kidney After Trauma

The traumatized organ is enlarged and a subcapsular haemorrhage appears as an echo-poor area, well distinguishable from the parenchyma. The same is true for injuries in the hilar region (Hofmann 1981).

Patients

At present we are treating 84 children with solitary kidneys on an outpatient basis. From 1979 to 1984, 30 of these patients ranging in age from 0 to 14 years were operated on for various urological diseases. Seventy-five percent had congenital solitary kidneys, two of which had been diagnosed prenatally.

Table 2 shows the various entities and the order of diagnostic steps. The children were referred to us because of failure to thrive, fever of unknown origin, urinary infections or enuresis. Tentative diagnosis was made by ultrasound and verified by further diagnostic steps (Table 3).

Following surgery of the ureter or kidney in patients with solitary kidney, assessment of urinary flow is of particular importance in the early postoperative phase as well as in the long-term follow-up.

Postoperative Course Following Pyeloplasty ($n = 14$)

In all children with hydronephrosis due to obstruction of the ureteropelvic junction we carried out an Anderson-Hynes pyeloplasty assessing the postoperative course sonographically in all cases. Since a transrenal splint is inserted into the ureter during the operation, an examination of urinary drainage is useful only after removal of the splint (i.e. on the 8th day postoperatively). The first sonographical examination of urinary drainage is carried out on the 14th day postoperatively; this is followed by monthly examinations for up to 1 year and thereafter every half year in the outpatient department.

An objective sonographical judgement of urinary drainage is possible only if the operative report is known. It must be taken into account that the dilatation of the renal collecting system caused by obstruction is irreversible in most cases. Thus, this intrarenal dilatation must be considered normal postoperatively. Besides the routine examination, we perform forced-diuresis sonography 1 year after surgery to assess the postoperative results.

Table 3. Pre- and postoperative diagnosis in paediatric surgical diseases of the solitary kidney

Disease	n	Primary diagnosis	Treatment	Postoperative diagnosis
Stenosis of the uretero-pelvic junction	14	1) Ultrasound 2) i.v. Pyelogram 3) Forced-diuresis sonography 4) Antegrade pyelogram	Anderson-Hynes pyeloplasty	1) Sonographic follow-up 2) Forced-diuresis sonography
Ostial stenosis	4	1) Ultrasound 2) i.v. Pyelogram 3) Forced-diuresis sonography 4) Voiding sono-cystography (VSC) 5) Cystoscopy	Leadbetter-Politano reimplantation	1) Sonographic follow-up 2) Voiding sono-cystography (VSC)
VUR without subvesical obstruction	5	1) Ultrasound 2) i.v. Pyelogram 3) Voiding sono-cystography + MCU	Leadbetter-Politano reimplantation	1) Sonographic follow-up 2) VSC
VUR with subvesical obstruction	5	1) Ultrasound 2) i.v. Pyelogram 3) VSC/MCU 4) Cystoscopy	1) Bouginage 2) Leadbetter-Politano reimplantation	1) Sonographic 2) VSC
Urolithiasis	2	1) Ultrasound 2) Forced-diuresis sonography	Pyelolithotomy	Sonographic follow-up

VSC, Voiding sonocystography; *MCU*, micturition cystourethrography

Because of transitory obstruction, we had to establish a temporary percutaneous nephrostomy for urinary drainage in one of our patients.

Forced-diuresis sonography performed 1 year after surgery in all patients showed still-delayed urinary transport but no obstruction.

Postoperative Course Following Reimplantation of the ureter into the Bladder ($n = 14$)

We applied the reimplantation technique of Politano and Leadbetter for patients with a VUR or an ostial stenosis. Sonographical control of urinary drainage is carried out on the 14th and 30th days following the antireflux operation, then monthly up to 1 year and every half year thereafter in the outpatient department. Sonographical examination includes the kidney, the ureter, and its vesical junction since obstructions occur primarily in this region.

Our experience shows that a stage-III DUT is normal in the early postoperative phase. Subsequently, the further development of the DUT is monitored. Radiological diagnosis is indicated only if the DUT shows progression or if there is still a stage-III DUT after 1 year.

Problems arose in children with ostial stenoses. In all cases there was kinking of the ureter to various degrees in addition to megalo-ureter. Twice we tried primary reimplantation according to Politano and Leadbetter alone, but this was followed by obstruction in the early postoperative phase. Urinary drainage returned to normal slowly following temporary percutaneous nephrostomy. For this reason we performed the reimplantation along with a protective Sober-plasty in two other children, with good results. The Sober ureterostomy was closed 6 months later in both cases.

We ran into similar, though minor, problems in solitary kidney patients with stage-IV VUR ($n = 4$). Our experience shows that the younger the patient, the slower the urinary drainage normalizes and the higher the reflux stage is. The question arises whether reimplantation in connection with a protective Sober ureterostomy might also be useful in stage-IV VUR with a predamaged solitary kidney. We have performed this in only one case, with good results.

Follow-up has revealed no stenoses so far. All 14 patients underwent control VSC 6 months following reimplantation without any signs of reflux recurrency.

Postoperative Course Following Pyelolithotomy ($n = 2$)

Following pyelolithotomy, we perform frequent postoperative control sonography in the outpatient department. Neither during the early postoperative phase nor in the long-term follow-up have we found evidence of pathological conditions such as residual calculi.

Discussion

The frequency of renal disease or life-threatening complications in patients with solitary kidney makes special care for these children necessary. Obviously, we have to revise our former opinion of an unrestricted life expectancy for such patients, as well as our tendency to often conservative treatment of diseased solitary kidneys. Appropriate therapy is determined exclusively by the quality of diagnostic methods. Diagnostic techniques hitherto in use are invasive and burdened with radiation exposure. Moreover, follow-up examinations must be performed frequently in a diseased solitary kidney. Sonography has the great advantage of allowing continuous non-invasive control of the solitary kidney and the urinary tract. The subtle morphological diagnosis makes it possible to detect even minor norm variants (i.e. stage-I DUT, which is typically found in an ampullary pelvis). A subtle differentiation of the parenchymal echo texture renders a distinction between acute and chronic diseases possible. However, renal function can be assessed only indirectly, requiring an i.v. pyelogram in any case. For further diagnosis, however, sonographical methods should be applied primarily, giving the indication for invasive methods in individual cases. The sonographical function tests described above provide a very good primary diagnosis. FDU, for instance, is an excellent tool for the differentiation of DUT under physiological conditions and of obstructive and non-obstructive uropathies without radiation exposure and invasive techniques. The same is true for reflux diagnosis, where sonography is the first diagnostic choice, since even a slight ascent of bladder contents to the solitary kidney can be disclosed.

In our opinion, there are at present three main indications for sonography in the treatment of solitary kidneys:

1. Continuous sonographical control of the solitary kidney for early detection of pathological changes. Thereafter, individual application of sonographical function tests. If an indication for surgery is derived from these methods, radiological techniques must be individually applied.
2. Follow-up examinations in already diagnosed and conservatively treated diseases of solitary kidneys, disclosing improvement, deterioration or unchanged findings after a certain time.
3. Follow-up examinations following surgery of the solitary kidney or the urinary tract, providing, in addition to an evaluation of urinary drainage, an assessment of renal growth, parenchymal development and echo texture. Operative long-term results can be verified by means of sonography. Early postoperative complications can be detected sonographically and treated.

In our experience, prenatal ultrasound and postnatal sonographical screening provide early detection of solitary kidneys and early treatment before clinical manifestation of damage to the kidney. Besides the early diagnosis of pathological changes, an extensive application of ultrasound renders possible a more individual application of invasive methods than has been the case hitherto, thus reducing radiation exposure of this region near the gonads. The possibility of early active surgical intervention raises hopes for a better life expectancy of children with solitary kidney.

References

Beyer H-J (1984) Sonografische Kontrolle der Abflußverhältnisse nach Antirefluxoperationen. Dissertation, Martin-Luther-University, Halle
Beyer H-J (1985) Prae- und postoperative sonografische Diagnostik beim vesico-ureteralen Reflux im Kindesalter. Thesis, MLU, Halle
Beyer H-J, Hofmann V (1985a) Sonografische Beurteilung der Abflußverhältnisse nach Antirefluxoperationen im Kindesalter. Z Urol Nephrol 78:17
Beyer H-J, Hofmann V (1985b) Das Miktionssonourogramm: eine neue Methode zur Erfassung des vesico-ureteralen Refluxes. Ultraschall 6:182
Brod J (1964) Die Nieren. Volk und Gesundheit, Berlin
Dinkel E, Peters H, Dittrich M (1982) Sonografische Diagnostik der Harntransportstörungen. Ultraschall Med 4:87

Fida B (1960) Minerva Med 30:1300
Fukala E, Fritz W (1976) Kinder mit Einzelnieren — eine Risikogruppe. Kipra 7:301
Hofmann V (1981) Ultraschall (B-scan) im Kindesalter. Thieme, Leipzig
Hofmann W, Forth H-J (1981) Erkrankungen von Einzelnieren. Z Urol Nephrol 74:75
Rockstroh H (1967) Das Lebensschicksal der Einnierigen. Volk und Gesundheit, Berlin
Rockstroh H, Samtleben W (1974) Die kompensatorische Hypertrophie der Restniere. Z Urol 67:931
Stojkovio J, Payer J, Siman J (1972) Effect on renal blood flow of unilateral nephrectomy and gradual damping of the abdominal aorta distal from the renal arteries. Int Urol Nephrol 4:407
Williams DI (1974) Urology in childhood. In: Andersson L, Gittes RF, Goodwin WE, Lutzeyer W, Zingg E (eds) Encyclopedia of urology. Springer, Berlin Heidelberg New York

Renal Function in Single-Kidney Rats

A. P. Provoost, M. H. De Keijzer, J. N. Wessel, and J. C. Molenaar

Summary

Can a single kidney survive for a normal life span? This is the type of question frequently asked by patients and especially by parents of children who lose one kidney in early childhood. Based on our wide experience with single-kidney rats, we will try to give an answer to this question. After the removal of its counterpart, the single remaining kidney will rapidly adapt to the new situation by a compensatory increase in the glomerular filtration rate (GFR) and renal mass. This is true not only for intact kidneys but also for damaged ones. The GFR level obtained by damaged kidneys will be less than that of intact single kidneys, however, depending on the degree of initial damage. The GFR is stable for a certain period of time, which is longer for intact single kidneys than for damaged kidneys and also depends on the daily protein intake; after that renal function will deteriorate. This decline in GFR is preceded by a marked increase in urinary protein excretion. Although the follow-up period is not completed yet, the survival time of single intact kidneys in rats on a normal diet is expected to be 15%–20% less than the normal rat life span. In rats on a lifelong high protein intake the kidney survival time drops to 40% below the normal rat life span. In rats on a moderately reduced protein intake, however, single intact kidneys may survive for a normal life span. The situation is worse for single damaged kidneys. Depending on the severity of the initial damage, kidney survival time will be much less than a normal life span. We studied rats with an initial recovery to 75% of renal function. Despite this initial recovery, the animals died of renal failure within 50% of the expected life span. A low-protein diet prolonged the renal survival by about 12%, a high-protein diet shortened it by the same percentage.

Zusammenfassung

Kann eine Einzelniere ein Leben lang zufriedenstellend funktionieren? Diese Frage wird uns sehr häufig gestellt, besonders oft von den Eltern der Kinder, die in früher Kindheit eine Niere verloren haben. Wir haben sehr viele Versuche an Ratten mit einer Einzelniere durchgeführt und wir wollen versuchen, diese Frage zu beantworten. Nach dem Entfernen einer Niere paßt sich die übriggebliebene

Department of Pediatric Surgery, Erasmus University, P. O. Box 1738, 3000 DR Rotterdam, The Netherlands

Progress in Pediatric Surgery, Vol. 23
Ed. by L. Spitz et al.

Niere sehr schnell der neuen Situation an und kompensiert durch Erhöhung der Glomerulumfiltrationsrate und der Nierenmasse. Dies trifft nicht nur bei gesunden Nieren, sondern auch bei geschädigten zu. Die Glomerulumfiltrationsrate ist jedoch niedriger bei geschädigten als bei gesunden Einzelnieren und hängt von dem Grad der Schädigung ab. Sie bleibt eine Zeitlang unverändert (länger bei gesunden Einzelnieren als bei geschädigten) und hängt auch mit der täglichen Proteinzufuhr zusammen. Danach verschlechtert sich die Nierenfunktion. Der Verringerung des Glomerulumfiltrats geht eine deutliche Proteinurie voraus. Obwohl die Versuchstiere weiterhin beobachtet werden, kann man erwarten, daß die Lebensdauer der gesunden Einzelniere um 15% bis 20% kürzer als die durchschnittliche Lebenszeit der Ratte sein wird. Bei Ratten, die ihr Leben lang eine proteinreiche Nahrung erhalten haben, bleibt die Lebensdauer der Niere sogar um 40% unter der durchschnittlichen Lebenszeit. Bei Ratten, die eine leicht reduzierte Proteinzufuhr erhalten haben, kann jedoch die Niere während der ganzen Lebenszeit funktionieren. Die Situation ist noch ernster bei geschädigten Einzelnieren. Je nachdem, wie schwer die ursprüngliche Schädigung ist, wird die Niere nur während eines Bruchteils der durchschnittlichen Lebensdauer funktionieren. Wir haben Ratten beobachtet, die zuerst 75% der Nierenfunktion wiedererlangt hatten und dennoch während der ersten Hälfte der durchschnittlichen Lebensdauer starben. Eine proteinarme Diät verlängert diese Zeit um ca. 12% und eine proteinreiche Diät verkürzt sie entsprechend.

Résumé

Combien de temps peut-on survivre avec un seul rein? C'est une question que nos patients nous posent fréquemment et plus souvent encore les parents des enfants ayant perdu un rein dans leur petite enfance. Nous avons pratiqué un grand nombre d'expériences sur des rats avec un rein unique et nous sommes en mesure d'essayer de répondre à cette question. Nous avons constaté qu'après l'ablation d'un rein, celui qui reste en place s'adapte très rapidement à la nouvelle situation qu'il compense par augmentation du taux de filtration glomérulaire et de la masse rénale. Ceci se produit non seulement dans le cas des reins sains mais aussi dans le cas des reins pathologiques. Il va de soi que le taux de filtration atteint par un rein pathologique reste inférieur à celui d'un rein unique sain et dépendra de l'ampleur de la lésion initiale. Le taux de filtration reste stable pendant un certain temps (ce laps de temps étant plus long pour le rein unique sain que pour le rein unique pathologique) et on notera que ce taux de filtration est étroitement lié à l'apport quotidien en protéines, puis la fonction rénale ira en se détériorant. Cette détérioration de la fonction rénale est précédée par une nette augmentation de la protéinurie. La poursuite de l'expérience sous surveillance confirme le fait que le rein unique des rats ayant un régime alimentaire normal continue à fonctionner pendant un laps de temps inférieur de 15%–20% à la durée moyenne théorique de la vie. Chez les rats ayant un régime hyperprotéique durant toute leur vie, la période de fonctionnement du rein unique sera de 40% inférieure à la durée normale de la vie du rat. Chez les rats ayant un régime dans lequel on a modérément réduit l'apport en protéines, un rein unique intact peut fonctionner durant toute la durée de la vie moyenne théorique. La situation sera encore plus grave quand le rein unique est pathologique. Selon la gravité de la lésion initiale, le rein ne fonctionnera que sur une période de temps nettement inférieure à la durée moyenne de la vie théorique. Nous avons suivi des rats présentant initialement une récupération atteignant 75% et qui pourtant sont morts par insuffisance né-phrétique durant la première moitié de la durée de vie théorique. Un régime pauvre en protéines prolonge cette survie de 12% environ et un régime riche en protéines l'écourte d'autant.

Introduction

It has long been recognized that animals as well as human beings born with a single kidney may lead quite normal lives (for historical reviews on this subject see Nowinsky 1969 and Peters 1979). Since the first planned unilateral nephrectomy (UNX) in 1869, this type of operation has frequently been performed. In fact, the whole concept of renal transplantation, as well as the use of living kidney donors, is based on the principle that a single kidney will suffice to sustain life. Both surgeons and physicians have become familiar with the compensatory enlargement of the remaining kidney. A concept was developed in the 1880s explaining the events following the loss of renal mass, based on the idea that urine formation was a process of renal secretion of water and solutes. According to this concept the single remaining kidney has to secrete more water and solutes and thus has to work harder. This concept had to be abandoned when new explanations for the formation of urine were developed around 1910 and firmly established in the 1930s. Urine is the ultimate result of a high rate of glomerular filtration and an almost equally high rate of tubular reabsorption of water and vital solutes. When it became possible to measure the glomerular filtration rate (GFR), it was soon shown that after UNX the GFR of the remaining kidney increased to about 70%–80% of that of the previous two-kidney value. This compensatory hyperfiltration diminishes the adverse effects of UNX. A detailed review of the functional aspects of a decrease in renal mass by Hayslett appeared in 1979. A growing body of evidence suggests that the increased GFR of the remaining nephrons and the hemodynamical changes involved in the compensation process may have pathological consequences in the long run (Brenner 1985). Surgeons, especially pediatric surgeons and urologists, are frequently asked by patients and parents, "Can one live with a single kidney?" and more specifically, "Can one live a normal life?" and "Can a single kidney, intact or possibly even damaged, survive for a normal human life span of 70–75 years?"

In the present article we review our 10-year experience with the functional aspects of single-kidney rats. This review will include published as well as unpublished data concerning intact and damaged single kidneys of either adult or young rats, in comparison with results reported by other workers.

For the quantification of the GFR we used a method we developed on the basis of a publication by Layzell and Miller (1975), and which we have described in various articles (Provoost and Molenaar 1980a; Provoost et al. 1982, 1983). It uses the plasma clearance of chromium 51-labelled EDTA as a measure of the GFR. In short, a known amount of ^{51}Cr-labelled EDTA is injected intravenously. After 60 min a blood sample is drawn and the ^{51}Cr-labelled EDTA clearance is calculated with a formula based on volume of distribution of the radiotracer. The number of perfused glomeruli were determined by direct counting after staining with Indian ink.

The Compensatory Response of Intact Kidneys

Age-related Differences

A relationship between the degree of renal compensatory hypertrophy and age was suggested 60 years ago by Jackson and Shield (1927). When studying the compensatory changes in unilaterally nephrectomized immature rats, one has to differentiate between the normal and the compensatory growth of the kidney. The rat is born with rather immature kidneys after a gestation period of only 21 days; nephrogenesis continues after birth. The time required for the completion of nephrogenesis is now established to be 7–8 days (Larsson 1975; Larsson et al. 1980), though earlier studies reported nephrogenesis up to the age of 3 weeks (Arataki 1928). The nephrons develop in a centrifugal way. The most mature nephrons are in the juxtamedullary region, while the most immature are found in the superficial renal cortex. Based on studies done during the mid 1960s of the RNA, DNA, and total protein content in the normal growing kidney, the renal growth cycle in the rat has been divided into three phases (Winick and Noble 1965). The first phase extends from birth to about day 14 and consists mainly of hyperplasia. During the second phase, which extends until about day 40, renal growth occurs by a combination of hyperplasia and hypertrophy. The third phase after day 40 is characterized by hypertrophy. This concept was later challenged based on observations that cell multiplication continued during the period of rapid body growth, i.e. up to day 80–90 (Sands et al. 1979; Celsi et al. 1986). Thus, the third phase can be considered an extension of the second period, during which the contribution of hyperplasia slowly diminishes.

The functional development of the growing kidney is well established. Shortly after birth, the GFR is low for body weight (Falk 1955) as well as for kidney weight (Horster and Lewy 1970). In the 3-day-old rat the GFR is only 0.04 ml/min/g kidney weight, rising to about 0.3 ml/min/g kidney weight at an age of 16–18 days. Adult values for total and single-nephron GFR per gram of kidney weight were found in rats at an age of 6–7 weeks (Bengele and Solomon 1974; Aperia and Herin 1975; Provoost et al. 1983). From birth to about 7 weeks of age the increase in GFR outnumbers the increase in body weight. Consequently, the GFR per 100 g body weight increases from about 0.04 ml/min at an age of 3 days

Table 1. The compensatory response of glomerular filtration rate (GFR), the wet kidney weight (WKW), and the number of glomeruli after unilateral nephrectomy (UNX) in adult (13 weeks old) and weanling (3 weeks old) rats

	(n)	Body wt. (g)	GFR (ml/min/100 g)	WKW (mg/100 g)	Glomeruli (per kidney)
Adults					
Sham	(7)	430 ± 27	0.360 ± 0.012	343 ± 25	31.120 ± 1.007
UNX	(14)	429 ± 25	0.537 ± 0.058	491 ± 34	32.359 ± 2.659
UNX/sham (%)			149 ± 16	143 ± 10	104 ± 9
Weanling					
Sham	(9)	349 ± 30	0.385 ± 0.029	357 ± 24	33.071 ± 4.731
UNX	(12)	337 ± 31	0.630 ± 0.061	543 ± 44	32.611 ± 3.470
UNX/sham (%)			164 ± 16[a]	152 ± 12	99 ± 10

All data are mean ± S.D.

The GFR and WKW for sham-operated rats refer to only one-kidney values

[a] $P < 0.05$ when compared with adults (t-test)

(body wt. 10–15 g; Falk 1955) to a value of about 1.2 ml/min at an age of 6 weeks (body wt. about 120 g). From then on, the increase in body weight is greater than the increase in GFR, and consequently there is a drop in the GFR relative to body weight.

Various research groups have studied the effect of the normal development on compensatory renal response after UNX. Two questions have been raised. Firstly, is there an increase in the number of nephrons in (very) young rats after UNX? Secondly, is there a difference in the rate or the level of compensatory increase in the GFR?

The first question, after being studied between 1880 and 1930 (see Bonvalet 1979 for references), was raised again when various reports published in the 1970s indicated that there was an induction of new nephrons in the remaining kidneys of young rats nephrectomized at an age as late as the 48th day of life (Imbert et al. 1974; Canter and Goss 1975; Bonvalet 1979). During our studies in rats after UNX at an age of 3 or 13 weeks, we did not observe a difference in the number of glomeruli of the remaining kidneys compared with intact kidneys of sham-operated two-kidney control rats (Table 1). Furthermore, two other studies did not show any involvement of the formation of new nephrons in the compensatory changes in newborn rats after UNX (Kaufman et al. 1975; Larsson et al. 1980). Therefore, we can safely rule out the hypothesis of nephron induction in single kidneys of young rats after UNX.

Various experiments have been performed to determine whether the compensatory response of the remaining kidney after UNX differed between immature and adult animals. Earlier reports suggested that the compensatory response in renal mass was greater in young rats (Jackson and Shields 1927; Arataki 1928). More recent studies have confirmed and extended these findings. In 5-day-old rats the rate and extent of the compensatory growth after UNX was greater than in adult rats (Dicker and Shirley 1973; Celsi et al. 1986). It was also estimated (by the change in RNA/DNA ratio, or by the lack of change in protein/DNA ratio) that the degree of cortical cellular hypertrophy in young rats was smaller than in adults. Thus, it appears that in newborn rats, in contrast to adult rats, a significant contribution to the compensatory increase in renal mass comes from cellular hyperplasia. When the operation was performed at an age of 12 days (Larsson et al. 1980) or 3 weeks (Kaufman et al. 1975a) the extent of the compensatory increase in renal mass after UNX was also larger than that found in adult rats (Table 1). As with the compensatory increase in renal mass, the functional response of the kidney remaining after UNX in young rats appears greater than that observed in adult rats. In agreement with the results of other workers (Kaufman et al. 1975a; Larsson et al. 1980), our studies indicated that after UNX in rats up to 3 weeks of age the GFR of the remaining kidney increases more than in adult rats (Table 1).

In conclusion, in immature rats the compensatory response of the remaining kidney after UNX is enhanced when compared with that of adult rats. This enhanced response involves renal function as well as renal growth, but not the induction of new nephrons.

Compensatory Changes in GFR

The time course of the compensatory changes can be divided into three periods: (a) the acute changes during the first postoperative week; (b) the intermediate changes occurring from 1 week up to 3 months after the operation; and (c) the chronic changes in renal function of single kidneys developing more than 3 months after nephrectomy.

Acute. As early as 4 h after the removal of one kidney we found that the GFR of the remaining kidney had increased from 50% to approximately 65% of that of sham-operated control rats with two normal kidneys (Provoost and Molenaar 1980a). The level of the GFR remained almost constant during the first 48 h after UNX. The reports in the literature of an immediate increase in the GFR after UNX are markedly divergent. Shirley and Skinner (1978) demonstrated a 15% increase in the GFR and the ERPF within 150 min after UNX. Others, however, reported no changes up to 3 h after UNX (Peters 1963; Katz and Epstein 1967). An increase in the GFR 18–24 h after UNX has been reported by several other workers (Peters 1963; Dicker and Shirley 1971; Potter et al. 1972). At 48 h after UNX an increase in both total-kidney and single-nephron GFR has also been reported (Lopez-Novoa et al. 1982). This increase in GFR was accompanied by an increase in renal plasma flow, a decreased renal vascular resistance, and a hyperdynamic circulatory state with increased cardiac output and decreased total peripheral resistance. Total renal blood flow of the remaining kidney measured with microspheres 120 min after UNX rose by 180%. This renal vasodilatation is probably mediated by prostaglandins, since it was completely prevented by pretreatment with indomethacin (Hahne et al. 1985).

Intermediate. Between 1 and 4 weeks after UNX there is a slow further increase in the GFR of the remaining kidney. This increase in the GFR is at its maximum 2–4 weeks after UNX, when the GFR reaches a level 75%–80% of that of two healthy kidneys (Peters 1963; Katz and Epstein 1967; Dicker and Shirley 1971; Provoost and Molenaar 1980a). The rise in renal blood or plasma flow has been reported to exceed the change in GFR resulting in a fall in filtration fraction (Kaufman et al. 1975b; Finn 1982; Provoost et al. 1984a, b).

Micropuncture studies have delved more deeply into the mechanisms of the increase in the GFR. At the nephron level, the GFR is governed on the one hand by a pressure difference, due to the imbalance between transcapillary hydraulic and colloid osmotic pressures, and on the other hand by the ultrafiltration coefficient, K_f, which expresses the physical characteristics of the filtration membrane. K_f is equal to the product of the hydraulic permeability and the area of the capillary filtering surface (Brenner and Humes 1977; Tucker and Blantz 1977). After UNX, an increase in the single-nephron GFR was initially reported to result primarily from a higher transcapillary pressure gradient, i.e. a glomerular hypertension, without a change in K_f (Deen et al. 1974). However, this has not been firmly established. Finn (1982) reported that 2 weeks after UNX single-nephron GFR and glomerular plasma flow had increased. The estimated glomerular hydrostatic pressure remained the same, but K_f was increased by 36%. Indirect evidence for an increase in K_f stems from morphometric analyses of the renal corpuscule during hypertrophy. At least two groups (Olivetti et al. 1980; Seyer-Hansen et al. 1985) reported an increase in the filtration surface area. This increase, however, was not sufficient to completely explain the increase in GFR after UNX.

The compensatory response of the remaining kidney in rats appears to be completed within 4 weeks after UNX. Between 4 weeks and 3 months after UNX we have observed very little change in either the GFR or the ERPF. Both functional parameters remain constant during this period (Provoost et al. 1982, 1984a; De-Keijzer et al. 1984).

Chronic. Since it minimizes the decrease in total GFR, hyperfiltration of the kidney that remains after UNX has generally been regarded as beneficial. However, experiments in rats with a more severe reduction in the number of nephrons (>80%) demonstrated an early destruction of the remnant glomeruli (Shimamura and Morrison 1975). Consequently, we may ask whether initially intact single kidneys remaining after UNX are in the long run also subjected to a deterioration in function. Such a slow deterioration was at least suggested by some studies of the long-term effects of UNX in human kidney donors. Studies performed in kidney donors more than 10 years after UNX showed a higher incidence of proteinuria and hypertension as compared with their pre-UNX values and matched control subjects (Hakim et al. 1984). Other studies, however, showed little or no adverse

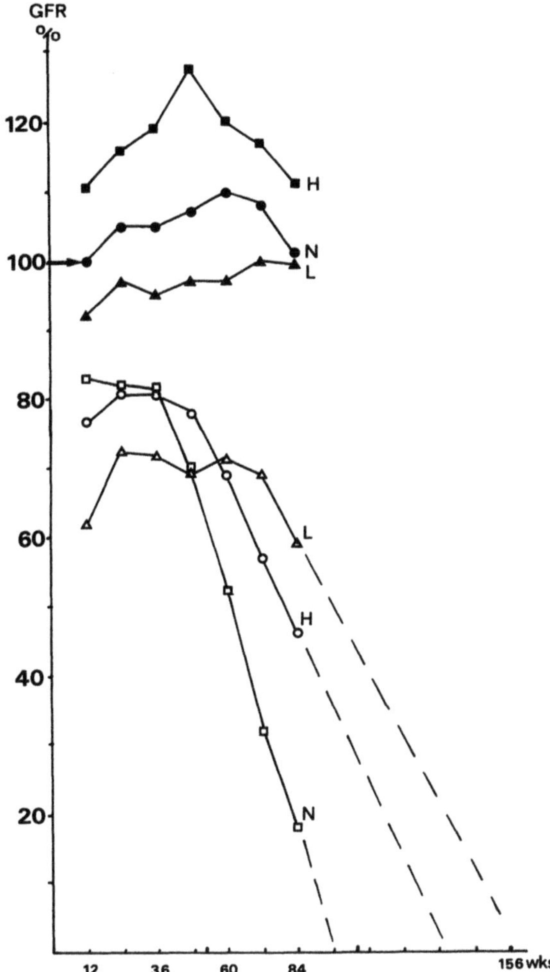

Fig. 1. Longitudinal changes in the glomerular filtration rate *(GFR)* of two-kidney and UNX rats on a normal *(N)*, high-*(H)*, or low-*(L)* protein diet during an 84-week follow-up period. Data are given as means and represent the GFR in ml/min as a percentage of the two-kidney value at week 12 *(arrow)*, being 2.072 ml/min. *Solid symbols,* two-kidney rats; *open symbols,* UNX rats; *circles,* normal diet; *squares,* high-protein diet; *triangles,* low-protein diet

effects of kidney donation after 10–20 years of compensatory hyperfiltration (Weiland et al. 1984; Anderson et al. 1985a). Consequently, UNX in living kidney donors may still be regarded as safe and ethically justified (Sutherland 1985; Sterioff 1985). Studies in patients nephrectomized for renal disease (Kiprov et al. 1982; Zuchelli et al. 1983; Smith et al. 1985) showed proteinuria and focal glomeruloscerlosis in only some cases. However, patients with unilateral renal agenesis are more likely to develop focal glomerulosclerosis and renal failure (Kiprov et al. 1982; Thorner et al. 1984).

In man the development of these renal alterations apparently takes a very long period of time, on the order of 30%–50% of the normal life span. Consequently, to obtain early indications it may be useful to study rats with a normal life span of

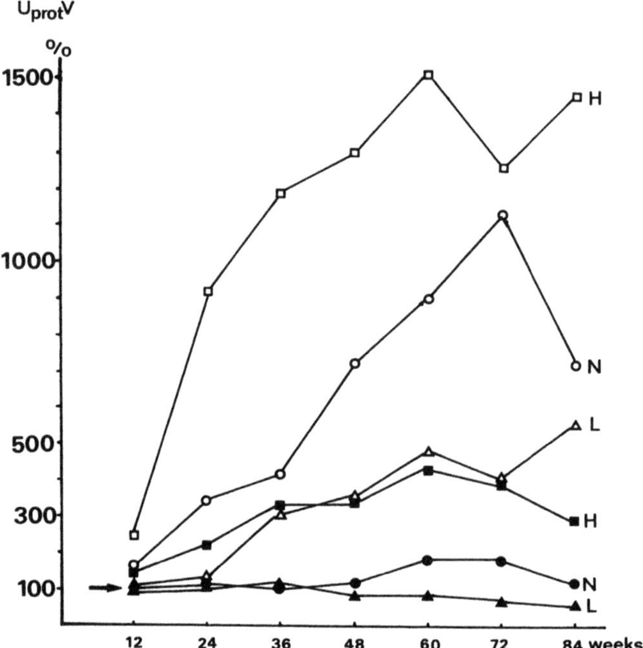

Fig. 2. Longitudinal changes in the urinary excretion of total protein $(U_{prot}V)$ of two-kidney and UNX rats on a normal (N), high-(H), or low-(L) protein diet during an 84-week follow-up period. Data are given as means and represent the $U_{prot}V$ in mg/24 h as a percentage of the two-kidney value at week 12 *(arrow)*, being 21.9 mg/24 h. *Solid symbols,* two-kidney rats; *open symbols,* UNX rats; *circles,* normal diet; *squares,* high-protein diet; *triangles,* low-protein diet

about 3 years (Burek 1978). Aging rats with two intact kidneys may develop renal lesions spontaneously. These changes consist of proteinuria and glomerular changes resembling focal glomerulosclerosis in human beings. Differences exist between various rat strains, and females of all strains appear to be less susceptible than males (Couser and Stilmant 1975; Elema and Arends 1975; Bolton et al. 1976; Kreisberg and Karnovsky 1978). Studies performed in rats more than 3 months after UNX have revealed that these animals are more prone to develop these spontaneous renal lesions (Striker et al. 1969; Grond et al. 1982). Detailed studies into the longitudinal changes of renal function and proteinuria after UNX have not yet been reported.

In our laboratory the long-term effects of UNX on renal function in rats are currently under investigation. After UNX or a sham operation at the age of 4 weeks, groups of rats (consisting of 15–20 animals) had their GFR and ERPF determined every 12 weeks. At the same time, in smaller subgroups, we determined the urinary protein excretion $(U_{prot}V)$. Up till now (March 1986) the animals have been followed up for 84 weeks after operation, i.e. about 60% of the expected life span. From the data presented in Fig. 1, it is clear that the GFR of sham-operated two-kidney rats remained stable during the 84 weeks of follow-up.

The $U_{prot}V$ of two-kidney rats increased slightly after week 48 (Fig. 2). A decline in the GFR of two-kidney rats is anticipated in the near future. Results of a serial study in aging rats (Alt et al. 1980), as well as higher levels of plasma creatinine and the increasing number of sclerotic glomeruli found in another study (Couser and Stilmant 1975), suggest a fall in GFR around the end of the second year of life. In human beings the age-related changes in renal function are better documented (Rowe et al. 1976; Lindeman et al. 1984). Creatinine clearance remains stable for about 40 years of life and subsequently declines particularly after the sixth decade. In persons over 80 years old, the creatinine clearance is reduced to about 60% of that of subjects in their 4th decade.

In our study the GFR of UNX rats remained stable for only 48 weeks and subsequently started to decrease. This decrease was preceded by an increase in the $U_{prot}V$. By 48 weeks, i.e. before the GFR started to decline, proteinuria was over five times that of two-kidney rats. From the rate at which the GFR fell, we may extrapolate that the UNX rats on a normal protein intake will die of renal failure between 120 and 144 weeks, i.e. at about 80% of the expected life span (Fig. 1).

Three human counterparts of the rat model with a single intact kidney can be distinguished: (a) patients with unilateral renal agenesis, (b) patients in whom one kidney is removed for unilateral renal disease and (c) living kidney donors. All three types are presently being studied in increasing numbers. Patients with unilateral renal agenesis are more likely to develop focal glomerulosclerosis and even renal failure before the age of 40 (Kiprov et al. 1982; Thorner et al. 1984). In living kidney donors (Vincenti et al. 1983; Hakim et al. 1984; Weiland et al. 1984; C. F. Anderson et al. 1985) and adult patients nephrectomized for unilateral renal disease (Kiprov et al. 1982; Zuchelli et al. 1983; Smith et al. 1985) who were studied up to 30 years after nephrectomy gross alterations in renal function were scarce. The same appears true for patients who underwent unilateral nephrectomy in childhood (Simon et al. 1982; Robitaille et al. 1985) and were studied up to 33 years later. From our experimental data in UNX rats, where the GFR remained stable for over 30% of the life span, we might extrapolate that in human beings significant changes in the GFR of single intact kidneys are not to be expected until 25 years after nephrectomy.

Effects of Low or High Protein Intake on Renal Function in UNX Rats

From studies of long duration carried out in the 1920s it is generally known that diets rich in protein result in renal deterioration in rats with two intact kidneys (Moise and Smith 1927; Newburgh and Curtis 1928). When UNX rats are fed a high-potein diet, they are even more susceptible to degeneration and sclerosis of glomeruli than animals with two kidneys (Lalich et al. 1975). Protein restriction delayed the spontaneous renal lesions and the development of renal failure common in aging rats (Berg and Simms 1960).

Apart from our experimental studies of the long-term effects of UNX on renal function in rats, we have studied the effects of both a high and a low protein intake. Instead of the normal rat chow, containing 24% protein, rats were fed either a high-protein diet containing 36% protein or a low-protein diet containing 12% protein. In rats with two intact kidneys a high protein intake caused an increase in GFR when compared with rats on a normal protein diet. There is a tendency for the GFR to decrease, starting from week 48. In contrast, rats on a low-protein diet had a lower GFR. On this diet the GFR remained stable during the 84-week follow-up period (Fig. 1). The $U_{prot}V$ also depended on the daily protein intake. Rats on a high-protein diet excreted more, while rats on a low protein diet, from week 60, excreted less protein than rats on a normal diet (Fig. 2).

Variations in the daily protein intake also had a very marked effect on renal function and $U_{prot}V$ in UNX rats. In UNX rats on a high-protein diet, the GFR started to decrease as early as 36 weeks after the operation. In those on a low-protein diet the GFR remained stable for at least 72 weeks (Fig. 1). On both diets the $U_{prot}V$ of UNX rats was higher than that of two-kidney rats. With a high-protein diet the absolute level of proteinuria was markedly higher than with a low-protein diet (Fig. 2). From the rate at which the GFR fell, we may extrapolate that the life expectancy of UNX rats on a high-protein diet is only 96 weeks, i.e. about 60% of a normal rat life span. On a low-protein diet, UNX rats will probably live out their normal life span of 3 years.

Compensatory Response of Single Damaged Kidneys

As with intact kidneys, single damaged kidneys are capable of showing compensatory changes. The final level of renal function, however, is greatly influenced by the degree of initial damage. We have studied various single-kidney models in rats, in which a damaged kidney had to recover in the absence of an intact contralateral kidney. Initially, studies with a follow-up of up to 3 months were performed in rats with isogeneically transplanted kidneys (Provoost et al. 1982, 1984a) and in rats with single kidneys damaged either by renal ischaemia (J. N. Wessel and A. Provoost, 1983, unpublished) or ureteral obstruction (Provoost and Molenaar 1980b, 1981). At the moment we are studying the chronic effects of the latter two models as well as the influence of a variation in protein intake upon these chronic changes.

Isogeneically Transplanted Kidneys

Isogeneic transplantation of an adult donor kidney to an adult recipient resulted in a GFR of about 80% of that of an adult UNX rat. An already hyperfunctioning transplanted kidney, from a donor that had been unilaterally nephrectomized 4 weeks earlier, reached the same level of GFR as that of a normal transplant (Provoost et al. 1982). This indicates that about 20% of the renal funtion had been lost during and following the transplantation procedure. The GFR of transplanted kidneys remained stable during a 15-week follow-up period, without any sign of functional deterioration (Provoost et al. 1982, 1984a).

When kidneys are transplanted isogeneically between rats of various sizes, the renal function adapts to the size of the recipients. Kidneys transplanted from (very) young rats into adults show a rapid augmentation of the compensatory response. On the other hand, transplantation of adult donor kidneys into young recipients causes an attenuation of the compensatory change in renal function (Provoost et al. 1984a). A similar mechanism may be effective in pediatric renal transplantation. Adult donor kidneys transplanted into children appear to adapt to the body size of the child (Provoost et al. 1984b).

Single Kidneys After Ischaemic Damage

The combination of unilateral renal ischaemia and contralateral nephrectomy is a well-known experimental model for the assessment of renal recovery (Jablonski et al. 1983). Contralateral nephrectomy enhances the rate and the degree of recovery of the ischaemic kidney (Finn 1980). When compared with the recovery in the presence of an intact kidney, it appears that this is due to improved hemodynamic parameters. There is a higher renal blood flow and ultrafiltration pressure as a result of a reduction in total renal vasoconstriction, especially preglomerular, normally present at 24 h after the ischaemic insult (Finn et al. 1984). There also seems to be less intratubular obstruction, resulting in an increased number of functioning nephrons (Finn 1980).

In our experiments, adult rats survived unilateral renal ischaemia of up to 75 min concomitant with contralateral UNX. When measured immediately or 1 week after the ischaemia, there was an inverse relation between the GFR and the duration of the ischaemia. When studied 3 weeks after the ischaemic insult, the GFR had recovered to a level similar to that of UNX rats. However, in contrast to rats subjected to 30, 45 or 60 min of ischaemia, where we found no mortality due to renal failure, 50% of the animals ultimately did not survive after 75 min of unilateral ischaemia and contralateral UNX (Table 2).

An identical experiment performed in 3-week-old weanling rats indicated that in these young rats the recovery of the GFR after 60 or 75 min of ischaemia was faster than in adult rats. At the same time, after 75 min of ischaemia the survival rate of weanling rats (> 80%) was higher than that of adult rats. In other words, immature growing kidneys tolerate a period of renal ischaemia better than adult kidneys (Table 2).

A more extensive and permanent reduction in the GFR of single kidneys can be produced by longer (> 75 min) periods of renal ischaemia. Rats survive such long periods of ischaemia only if the contralateral UNX is postponed for at least 1 week.

From the data presented in Table 3 it is clear that after an ischaemic period lasting more than 75 min there was only a partial recovery of the GFR, while the number of perfused glomeruli was found to be reduced. However, the reduction

Table 2. Effects on glomerular filtration rate (GFR) and the number of glomeruli of various periods of unilateral renal ischaemia plus contralateral nephrectomy (NX) in adult (A) and weanling (W) rats

	GFR – weeks post NX									Number of glomeruli
		GFR-0		GFR-1		GFR-3		GFR-15		
Ischaemic time										
UNX										
A	(9)	100 ± 8	(9)	100 ± 10	(9)	100 ± 8	(9)	100 ± 8	(8)	100 ± 10
W	(7)	100 ± 19	(6)	100 ± 23	(6)	100 ± 16	(7)	100 ± 12	(6)	100 ± 14
45 Min										
A	(10)	32 ± 24	(10)	81 ± 17	(10)	98 ± 8	(10)	98 ± 8	(10)	98 ± 12
W	(7)	50 ± 26	(7)	94 ± 17	(7)	97 ± 11	(7)	103 ± 13	(6)	86 ± 10
60 Min										
A	(10)	8 ± 10	(10)	60 ± 21	(9)	98 ± 17	(8)	102 ± 18	(8)	89 ± 13
W	(7)	11 ± 6	(7)	101 ± 23	(7)	100 ± 9	(6)	93 ± 10	(6)	91 ± 17
75 Min										
A	(10)	0 ± 0	(6)	38 ± 31	(5)	83 ± 25	(5)	84 ± 33	(5)	81 ± 14
W	(8)	7 ± 9	(8)	91 ± 30	(8)	91 ± 19	(8)	94 ± 22	(8)	88 ± 19

All data are mean ± S.D.

The GFR is given in ml/min/100 g body wt. as a percentage of the UNX rats. The number of glomeruli is given as a percentage of that of intact kidneys in UNX rats

Table 3. Effects on glomerular filtration rate (GFR) and the number of glomeruli of various periods of unilateral renal ischaemia plus contralateral nephrectomy (NX) 1 week later in adult (A) and weanling (W) rats

	GFR – weeks post NX									Number of glomeruli
		GFR-0		GFR-1		GFR-3		GFR-15		
Ischaemic time										
UNX										
A	(10)	100 ± 7	(8)	100 ± 8	(8)	100 ± 7	(8)	100 ± 9	(6)	100 ± 6
W	(8)	100 ± 12	(8)	100 ± 24	(8)	100 ± 9	(8)	100 ± 9	(6)	100 ± 10
75 Min										
A	(10)	18 ± 8	(10)	62 ± 20	(8)	69 ± 15	(7)	76 ± 28	(5)	96 ± 16
W	(10)	54 ± 22	(10)	74 ± 17	(10)	75 ± 23	(10)	73 ± 22	(7)	73 ± 12
90 Min										
A	(9)	8 ± 7	(7)	43 ± 14	(7)	49 ± 16	(5)	42 ± 24	(3)	75 ± 17
W	(9)	36 ± 24	(9)	51 ± 21	(8)	52 ± 33	(6)	46 ± 44	(3)	79 ± 31
105 Min										
A	(11)	2 ± 2	(11)	26 ± 12	(9)	31 ± 14	(8)	28 ± 15	(5)	59 ± 9
W	(5)	17 ± 16	(5)	45 ± 18	(5)	47 ± 25	(5)	26 ± 25	(3)	51 ± 19

All data are mean ± S.D.

The GFR is given in ml/min/100 g body wt. as a percentage of the UNX rats. The number of glomeruli is given as a percentage of that of intact kidneys in UNX rats

in GFR was greater than the reduction in the number of perfused glomeruli. This means that the hyperfiltration of these remaining glomeruli is less than that of intact kidneys remaining after UNX. Dividing the GFR by the number of glomeruli shows that the mean nephron GFR of single kidneys damaged by 105 min of ischemia is only 48% of that of intact single kidneys. In this way, the ischaemically damaged single kidneys differ from single kidneys remaining after progressive surgical ablation. After removal of 75% of the renal mass, mean nephron GFR increased by about 150% (Kaufman et al. 1975b). This increase was much higher than that observed in intact kidneys remaining after UNX. Consequently, the mean nephron GFR of the glomeruli remaining after partial ablation increased to a level of about 150% of that of glomeruli of single intact kidneys.

Single Kidneys After Temporary Ureteral Obstruction

The degree of recovery of the GFR after a temporary complete unilateral ureteral obstruction in rats depends on the duration of the obstruction. In adult rats (Provoost and Molenaar 1981) as well as in weanling rats (A. P. Provoost, H. Visser, J. Setyo, 1984, unpublished data) we studied the recovery of the obstructed kidney either in the presence or in the absence of an intact contralateral kidney. When measured after 2 weeks of recovery, the GFR of single kidneys remaining after the removal of a ureteral obstruction lasting 1 week and contralateral UNX amounted to about 70% of that of intact single kidneys. With 2 weeks of ureteral obstruction the recovery was about 35% and with 3 weeks of obstruction it dropped to about 15% (Provoost and Molenaar 1981).

These data were confirmed in a subsequent experiment and expanded with data on the effects of temporary ureteral obstruction in weanling rats (Table 4). In weanling rats, the degree of recovery was about the same as that in adult rats after identical periods of ureteral obstruction. However, the mortality after 3 weeks of ureteral obstruction plus removal of the intact kidney was higher in weanling rats than in adults. Thus, immature kidneys appear to be more vulnerable to the damaging effect of ureteral obstruction. This is in contrast to the effects of temporary ischaemia, to which immature kidneys appear less vulnerable than adult kidneys. As with ischaemic damage, the reduction in GFR is greater than the reduction in the number of perfused glomeruli, and therefore the mean nephron GFR of these damaged kidneys will be less than that of intact single kidneys.

Chronic Changes in the GFR of Single Damaged Kidneys and the Influence of a Low and High Protein Intake

Partial removal of renal tissue from the kidney remaining after UNX enhances the development of glomerulosclerosis (Shimamura and Morrison 1975), normally occurring in intact single kidneys (Grond et al. 1982). In most of the recently pub-

Table 4. Effects on glomerular filtration rate (GFR) and the number of glomeruli of various periods of unilateral ureteral obstruction plus contralateral nephrectomy (NX) at the time of removal of the obstruction in adult (A) and weanling (W) rats

	GFR − weeks post NX								Number of glomeruli
	GFR-0		GFR-1		GFR-3		GFR-15		
Obstruction time									
UNX									
A	(7)	100 ± 6	(7)	100 ± 3	(7)	100 ± 3	(7)	100 ± 2	(7) 100 ± 10
W	(9)	100 ± 16	(9)	100 ± 6	(9)	100 ± 3	(7)	100 ± 6	(6) 100 ± 6
7 Days									
A	(9)	9 ± 2	(9)	65 ± 5	(8)	71 ± 6	(7)	71 ± 11	(5) 79 ± 14
W	(11)	10 ± 2	(7)	53 ± 6	(6)	68 ± 8	(5)	66 ± 15	(4) 77 ± 14
14 Days									
A	(11)	10 ± 2	(9)	28 ± 5	(8)	40 ± 27	(7)	44 ± 6	(4) 75 ± 10
W	(6)	11 ± 3	(3)	28 ± 13	(3)	44 ± 12	(2)	42 ± 1	(2) 62 ± 7
21 Days									
A	(8)	3 ± 2	(5)	6 ± 3	(4)	22 ± 2	(3)	24 ± 2	N.S.
W	(6)	2 ± 1		N.S.		N.S.		N.S.	N.S.

All data are mean ± S.D.

The GFR is given in ml/min/100 g body wt. as a percentage of the UNX rats. The number of glomeruli is given as a percentage of that of intact kidneys in UNX rats

lished experiments, renal parenchymal ablation is used as a standard model. The amount of renal tissue removed may vary from 1½ to 1⅚ of the two kidneys. Removal of 75% or more of the renal mass results in a syndrome of azotemia, proteinuria and arterial hypertension (Shimamura and Morrison 1975; Purkerson et al. 1976). After removal of such large amounts of renal tissue the adaptive responses of the remaining glomeruli more than doubles the single-nephron GFR (Kaufman et al. 1975; Hostetter et al. 1981) after 1–4 weeks. This marked increment is due to two factors. The single-nephron glomerular plasma flow is elevated along with the glomerular capillary pressure, resulting from striking vasodilatation of remnant intrarenal arterioles (Hostetter et al. 1981). Despite these adaptations limiting the fall in total GFR, the life span of the rats after subtotal nephrectomy is greatly reduced because of a continuous further deterioration of renal function (Kleinknecht et al. 1979; Salusky et al. 1981; El-Nahas et al. 1983; Louari et al. 1984; Kenner et al. 1985).

The rate of fall of the renal function and the mortality are further increased by feeding the animals a high-protein diet (Kleinknecht et al. 1979; Louari et al. 1984; Kenner et al. 1985). Other factors aggravating the renal dysfunction after renal mass reduction include hypertension (Tsuruda et al. 1986) and probably a high-sodium diet – i.e. at least in UNX rats (Lalich et al. 1975). The renal dysfunction can be diminished and the survival time of rats with a severe reduction in renal mass can be prolonged by a low-protein (Kleinknecht et al. 1979; Salusky et al. 1981; El-Nahas et al. 1983; Louari et al. 1984; Kenner et al. 1985), a low-phosphate (Ibels et al. 1978; Lumertgul et al. 1986), a high linoleic acid (Barcelli et al. 1982), or a low-sodium diet (Daniels and Hostetter 1986). A low-protein diet largely prevents the glomerular haemodynamic alterations leading to hyperfiltration (Hostetter et al. 1981). A better control of the systemic blood pressure (Jackson et al. 1986), more specifically control of glomerular hypertension, which may be achieved by the use of converting enzyme inhibitors (S. Anderson et al. 1985b) but not by all antihypertensive drugs (Anderson et al. 1986), ameliorates the proteinuria and glomerulosclerosis. Finally, anticoagulant drugs have proved to be beneficial (Purkerson et al. 1982; Olson 1984).

In experiments with progressive renal ablation, longitudinal measurements of changes in renal function have received little attention. Such measurements consisted mainly of serial determinations of serum creatinine and/or blood urea nitrogen levels (Kleinknecht et al. 1979; Salusky et al. 1981; El-Nahas et al. 1983). These levels, especially that of urea, are greatly affected by the composition of the diet and thus not very sensitive. Furthermore, experiments with models other than severe renal ablation, with less initial renal injury, were lacking. Consequently, we have initiated a lifelong study of the effects of a moderate inital renal damage on the regression of renal function. At the same time we are studying the influence of a high- and a low-protein diet on this process.

At this moment (March 1986), these experiments have been underway for 2 years. In combination with the two-kidney and UNX rats, already described above, two models of single damaged kidneys were used. They were produced either by a combination of 7 days of complete unilateral ureteral obstruction and

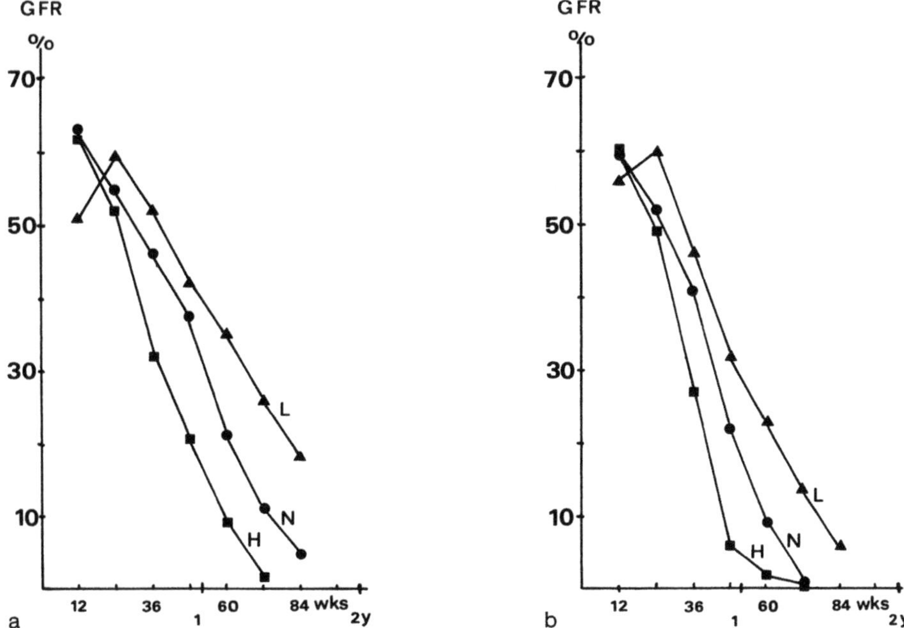

Fig. 3. a Longitudinal changes in the glomerular filtration rate *(GFR)* of single kidney rats damaged by temporary ischemia on a normal *(N)*, high-*(H)*, or low-*(L)* protein diet during an 84-week follow-up period. Data are given as means and represent the GFR in ml/min as a percentage of the two-kidney value at week 12, being 2.072 ml/min. *Circles,* normal diet; *squares,* high-protein diet; *triangles,* low-protein diet. **b** Longitudinal changes in the glomerular filtration rate *(GFR)* of single kidney rats damaged by temporary ureteral obstruction on a normal *(N)*, high-*(H)*, or low-*(L)* protein diet during an 84-week follow-up period. Data are given as means and represent the GFR in ml/min as a percentage of the two-kidney value at week 12, being 2.072 ml/min. *Circles,* normal diet; *squares,* high-protein diet; *triangles,* low-protein diet

UNX on the day of removal of the obstruction, or by a combination of 90 min of unilateral renal ischaemia and UNX 1 week later. The primary operations were carried out in weanling rats at an age of 3 weeks. After the operations the animals were placed on either a normal diet (24% protein), a high-protein (36%) diet, or a low-protein (12%) diet. Renal function was determined every 12 weeks. For analyses animals were selected on the basis of two criteria. Firstly, the single damaged kidneys had to show a good recovery with a GFR greater than 50% of that of UNX rats with single intact kidneys on the same diet. Secondly, only animals dying of end-stage renal failure were included. In this way, groups were created consisting of 15–20 rats, except for the group of rats with ischaemically damaged kidneys, which contained only 7 rats.

At the first measurement, i.e. 12 weeks after the operation, the GFR of the single damaged kidney was about 75% of that of intact single kidneys remaining after UNX (Fig. 3a, b). Thus, the initial recovery was good. However, during the follow-up period there was a steady decrease in the GFR. The rate of fall appeared to depend on the dietary protein intake as well as on the cause of the renal damage. The rate of fall of of the GFR was greater in kidneys damaged by ureteral obstruction than in those damaged by ischaemia. When compared with that in rats on a normal diet, the rate of fall was slightly less in those on a low-protein diet and slightly higher in those on a high-protein diet. The survival time of these rats with single damaged kidneys is drastically shortened. Almost all of the rats with single damaged kidneys on a normal diet died of renal failure within 1.5 years, half the normal life span. For rats on a low-protein diet the survival time was prolonged by about 20 weeks, i.e. about ⅛ of the normal life span. For those on a high-protein diet the survival time was shortened when compared with the normal diet, also by about 20 weeks.

All rats with single damaged kidneys had severe and progressive proteinuria. The daily protein excretion was higher on a high-protein diet and lower on a low-protein diet when compared with a normal diet. Single kidneys damaged by ischaemia lost less protein than those damaged by ureteral obstruction. For instance, rats with ischaemically damaged single kidneys at week 12 on a low-protein, normal, or high-protein diet had a daily protein excretion which was respectively 1.3, 3.2, and 4.4 times that of two-kidney rats on a normal diet. At week 36 these figures had increased to 5.7, 11.1, and 14.6 times that of rats with two intact kidneys on a normal diet.

In human beings there are many situations where only a single damaged kidney is present. In this connection, we should like to mention oligomeganephronia (McGraw et al. 1984) — although it usually presents bilaterally, solitary kidneys with ureteral abnormalities, patients with bilateral renal abnormalities in whom only the most severely affected kidney was removed, and long-surviving renal transplant recipients. These types of abnormalities constitute a highly increased risk for an early development of end-stage renal failure.

Mechanism(s) of the Regression of Renal Function of Single Kidneys

Based on experimental studies, Brenner and coworkers developed a comprehensive hypothesis in 1981 to account for the deterioration of renal function after the loss of renal mass (Hostetter et al. 1981). It was suggested "that the 'adaptive' increments in single-nephron GFR may represent a potentially adverse response...". It was not clear whether the hyperfiltration as such or some haemodynamic determinant thereof was responsible for the derangement. In later reviews this hypothesis was extended and modified (Brenner 1983, 1985; Brenner et al. 1982; Hostetter 1984; S. Anderson et al. 1985a), although it remained essentially the same. The adaptive renal vasodilation results in long-term elevations of glomerular capillary pressure and flow. These haemodynamic factors promote glomerular hyperfiltration, but they impair the permeability selective properties of the glomerular wall and very likely injure the component cells of the glomerulus. These alterations finally lead to glomerulosclerosis and a further deterioration of the filtration process.

Conclusion

In 1938, Deming stated that "urologists have all been asked by patients... 'Can I live with one kidney?' and 'What does the future have in store for me?'." More recently, these questions have been asked again with respect to the future of living related kidney donors. The answer to the first question is simple. Yes, one can live with a single kidney, either intact or damaged. What conclusions can we draw from the rat experiments concerning the future of people living with only one kidney? Of course, care has to be taken in extrapolating findings in rats to the human situation. Nevertheless, assuming that our findings also apply to human beings, we surmise that a single intact kidney cannot sustain the demands of a normal, 75-year human life span. On a normal protein intake, the GFR remained stable during one third of the life span. In human beings, then, a significant fall in the GFR could be expected after one had lived for over 25 years with an intact single kidney. On a normal diet the survival time of a single kidney will be reduced by 15%–20%. On a high daily protein intake the onset of renal deterioration is earlier and the rate is increased. Consequently, single intact kidneys on such a high protein intake survive only 60% of a normal life span, i.e. in human terms, 45 years. A moderate reduction of the daily protein load, however, may create a situation in which a single kidney can last a full normal life span.

People living with only one kidney most probably bear a somewhat greater risk of developing chronic renal failure within a normal life span than those with two intact kidneys. As the renal functional deterioration is a slow process, this risk is higher in the young than in the middle-aged or old. Functional deterioration in a predamaged single kidney has an earlier onset. Consequently, patients with bilateral renal abnormalities in whom the most damaged kidney is removed and children born with a single (normal or abnormal) kidney are special risk groups, for whom regular surveillance and appropriate therapeutic measures should be considered. The same holds true for long-term renal transplant recipients and, to a much lower degree, for kidney donors. Appropriate interventions may consist of dietary measures, a reduction of the intake of protein, phosphate, and sodium, and good blood pressure control with drugs that also prevent glomerular hypertension.

In case of single damaged kidneys the situation worsens. Even kidneys that had an initial recovery to about 75% that of single intact kidneys rapidly declined in function. The survival time of such kidneys is only 60% that of normal ones. In human beings, this would be 45 years. The onset of this decline can be slightly delayed and the rate of deterioration diminished by reducing the daily protein intake. On a moderate protein intake, in rats, the survival time is expected to increase by about 12% (in man, by 9 years). On the other hand, an increase in the daily protein intake accelerates renal deterioration and the survival time is reduced by 12%. If the initial damage is greater, however, the survival time of the single damaged kidney will be shorter. But even in this situation, therapeutic interventions may slow down the functional deterioration of the single kidney. Dietary restriction of protein, phosphate, and sodium, blood pressure control with drugs reducing the glomerular hypertension, and the use of anticoagulant drugs may be beneficial.

References

Alt JM, Hackbarth H, Deerberg F, Stolte H (1980) Proteinuria in rats in relation to age-dependent renal changes. Lab Animal 14:95–101

Anderson CF, Velosa JA, Frohnert PP, Torres VE, Offord KP, Vogel JP, Donadio JV Jr, Wilson DM (1985) The risks of unilateral nephrectomy: status of kidney donors 10 to 20 years postoperatively. Mayo Clin Proc 60:367–374

Anderson S, Meyer TW, Brenner BM (1985a) The role of hemodynamic factors in the initiation and progression of renal disease. J Urol 133:363–368

Anderson S, Meyer TW, Rennke HG, Brenner BM (1985b) Control of glomerular hypertension limits glomerular injury in rats with reduced renal mass. J Clin Invest 76:612–619

Anderson S, Rennke HG, Brenner BM (1986) In arresting progressive renal disease, all antihypertensive drugs are not created equal. Kidney Int 29:314

Aperia A, Herin P (1975) Development of glomerular perfusion rate and nephron filtration rate in rats 17–60 days old. Am J Physiol 228:1319–1325

Arataki M (1928) On the postnatal growth of the kidney, with special reference to the number and size of glomeruli (albino rat). Am J Anat 36:399–436

Barcelli UO, Weiss M, Pollak VE (1982) Effects of dietary prostaglandin presursor on the progression of experimentally induced chronic renal failure. J Lab Clin Med 100:786–797

Bengele HH, Solomon S (1974) Development of the renal response to blood volume expansion in the rat. Am J Physiol 237:364–368

Berg BN, Simms HS (1960) Nutrition and longevity in the rat. II. Longevity and the onset of disease with different levels of food intake. J Nutr 71:255–263

Bolton WK, Benton FR, Maclay JG, Sturgill BC (1976) Spontaneous glomerular sclerosis in aging Sprague-Dawley rats. Am J Pathol 85:277–300

Bonvalet JP (1979) Evidence of induction of new nephrons in immature kidneys undergoing hypertrophy. In: Peters G, Diezi J, Guignard J-P (eds) Renal adaptation to nephron loss. Karger, Basel, pp 73–77

Brenner BM (1983) Hemodynamically mediated glomerular injury and the progressive nature of kidney disease. Kidney Int 23:647–655

Brenner BM (1985) Nephron adaptation to renal injury or ablation. Am J Physiol 249:F324–F337

Brenner BM, Humes MD (1977) Mechanics of glomerular ultrafiltration. N Engl J Med 287:146–154

Brenner BM, Meyer TW, Hostetter TH (1982) Dietary protein intake and the progressive nature of kidney disease. N Engl J Med 307:652–660

Burek JD (1978) Pathology of aging rats. CRC, West Palm Beach, pp 21–27

Canter CE, Goss RJ (1975) Induction of extra nephrons in unilaterally nephrectomized immature rats. Proc Soc Exp Biol Med 148:294–296

Celsi G, Jakobsson B, Aperia A (1986) Influence of age on compensatory renal growth in rats. Pediatr Res 20:347–350

Couser WG, Stilmant MM (1975) Mesangial lesions and focal glomerular sclerosis in the aging rat. Lab Invest 33:491–501

Daniels BS, Hostetter TH (1986) Influence of dietary salt on chronic renal injury. Kidney Int 29:244

Deen WM, Maddox DA, Robertson CR, Brenner BM (1974) Dynamics of glomerular ultrafiltration in the rat. VII. Response to reduced renal mass. Am J Physiol 277:556–563

DeKeijzer MH, Provoost AP, Wolff ED, Kort WJ, Weijma IM, van Aken M, Molenaar JC (1984) The effect of a reduced sodium intake on postrenal transplantation hypertension in rats. Clin Sci 66:269–276

Deming CL (1938) The future of the unilaterally nephrectomized patient. J Urol 40:74

Dicker SE, Shirtley DG (1971) Mechanisms of compensatory renal hypertrophy. J Physiol (Lond) 219:507–523

Dicker SE, Shirley DG (1973) Compensatory renal growth after unilateral nephrectomy in the newborn rat. J Physiol (Lond) 228:193–202

El-Nahas AM, Paraskevakou H, Zoob S, Rees AJ, Evans DJ (1983) Effect of dietary protein restriction on the development of renal failure after subtotal nephrectomy in rats. Clin Sci 65: 399–406

Elema JD, Arends A (1975) Focal and segmental glomerular hyalinosis and sclerosis in the rat. Lab Invest 33:554–561

Falk G (1955) Maturation of renal function in infant rats. Am J Physiol 212:629–632

Finn WF (1980) Enhanced recovery from postischemic acute renal failure: micropuncture studies in the rat. Circ Res 46:440

Finn WF (1982) Compensatory renal hypertrophy in Spraque-Dawley rats. Glomerular ultrafiltration dynamics. Renal Physiol 5:222–234

Finn WF, Fernandez-Repollet E, Goldfarb D, Iaina A, Eliahou HE (1984) Attenuation of injury due to unilateral renal ischemia: delayed effects of contralateral nephrectomy. J Lab Clin Med 103:193–203

Grond J, Schilthuis MS, Koudstaal J, Elema JD (1982) Mesangial function and glomerular sclerosis in rats after unilateral nephrectomy. Kidney Int 22:338–343

Hahne B, Karlberg L, Persson AEG (1985) Renal vasodilatation after unilateral renal ablation. Ups J Med Sci 90:181–191

Hakim RM, Goldszer RC, Brenner BM (1984) Hypertension and proteinuria: long-term sequelae of uninephrectomy in humans. Kidney Int 25:930–936

Hayslett JP (1979) Functional adaptation to reduction in renal mass. Physiol Rev 59:137–163

Horster M, Lewy JE (1970) Filtration fraction and extraction of PAH during neonatal period in the rat. Am J Physiol 219:1061–1065

Hostetter TH (1984) Progressive glomerular injury: roles of dietary protein and compensatory hypertrophy. Pharmacol Rev 36:101S–107S

Hostetter TH, Olsen JL, Rennke HG, Venkatachalam MA, Brenner BM (1981) Hyperfiltration in remnant nephrons: a potentially adverse response to renal ablation. Am J Physiol 241: F85–F93

Ibels CS, Alfrey AC, Haut L, Huffer WE (1978) Preservation of function in experimental renal disease by dietary phosphate restriction. N Engl J Med 298:122–126

Imbert M, Berjal G, Moss N, de Rouffignac C, Bonvalet JP (1974) Number of nephrons in hypertrophic kidneys after unilateral nephrectomy in young and adult rats. A functional study. Pflugers Arch 346:279–290

Jablonski P, Howden PO, Rae DA, Birrell CS, Marshall VC, Tange J (1983) An experimental model for assessment of renal recovery from warm ischemia. Transplantation 35:198–204

Jackson B, Debrevi L, Cubela R, Whitty M, Johnston CI (1986) Renal function preservation by blood pressure reduction in the rat remnant kidney model of chronic renal failure (abstract). Kidney Int 29:320

Jackson CM, Shields M (1927) Compensatory hypertrophy of the kidney during various periods after unilateral nephrectomy in very young albino rats. Anat Rec 36:221–237

Katz AI, Epstein FH (1967) Relations of glomerular filtration and sodium reabsorption to kidney size in compensatory renal hypertrophy. Yale J Biol Med 40:222–230

Kaufman JM, Hardy R, Hayslett JP (1975a) Age-dependent characteristics of compensatory renal growth. Kidney Int 8:21–26

Kaufman JM, Siegel NJ, Hayslett JP (1975b) Functional and hemodynamic adaptation to progressive renal ablation. Circ Res 36:286–293

Kenner CH, Evan AP, Blomgren P, Aranoff GR, Luft FC (1985) Effect of protein intake on renal function and structure in partially nephrectomized rats. Kidney Int 27:739–750

Kiprov DD, Colvin RB, McCluskey RT (1982) Focal and segmental glomerulosclerosis and proteinuria associated with unilateral renal agenesis. Lab Invest 46:275–281

Kleinknecht C, Salusky I, Broyer M, Gubler M-C (1979) Effect of various protein diets on growth, renal function, and survival of uremic rats. Kidney Int 15:534–541

Kreisberg JI, Karnovsky MJ (1978) Focal glomerular sclerosis in the Fawn-Hooded rat. Am J Pathol 92:637–645

Lalich JJ, Burkholder PM, Paik WCW (1975) Protein overload nephropathy in rats with unilateral nephrectomy. Arch Pathol 99:72–79

Larsson L (1975) The ultrastructure of the developing proximal tubule in the rat kidney. J Ultrastruct Res 51:119–139

Larsson L, Aperia A, Wilton P (1980) Effect of normal development on compensatory renal growth. Kidney Int 18:29–35

Layzell D, Miller T (1975) Determination of the glomerular filtration rate in the rat using 51-Cr EDTA and a single blood sample. Invest Urol 13:200–204

Lindeman RD, Tobin JD, Shock NW (1984) Association between blood pressure and the rate of decline in renal function with age. Kidney Int 26:861–868

Lopez-Novoa JM, Ramos B, Martin-Oar JE, Hernando L (1982) Functional compensatory changes after unilateral nephrectomy in rats. General and intrarenal hemodynamic alterations. Renal Physiol 5:76–84

Louari D, Kleinknecht C, Gubler M-C, Broyer M (1984) Adverse effects of proteins on remnant kidney: dissociation from that of other nutrients. Kidney Int [Suppl 16] 24:S248–S253

Lumertgul D, Burke TJ, Gillum DM, Alfrey AC, Harris DC, Hammond WS, Schier RW (1986) Phosphate depletion arrests progression of chronic renal failure independent of protein intake. Kidney Int 29:658–666

McGraw M, Poucell S, Swett J, Baumal R (1984) The significance of focal segmental glomerulosclerosis in oligomeganephronia. Int J Pediatr Nephrol 5:67–72

Moise TS, Smith AH (1927) The effect of high protein diet on the kidneys. Arch Pathol 4:530–542

Newburgh LH, Curtis AC (1928) Production of renal injury in the white rat by the protein of the diet. Arch Intern Med 42:801–821

Nowinsky WW (1969) Early history of renal hypertrophy. In: Nowinsky WW, Goss RJ (eds) Compensatory renal hypertrophy. Academic, New York, pp 1–8

Olivetti G, Anversa P, Melissari M, Loud AV (1980) Morphometry of the renal corpuscle during postnatal growth and compensatory hypertrophy. Kidney Int 17:438–454

Olson JL (1984) Role of heparin as a protective agent following reduction of renal mass. Kidney Int 25:376–382

Peters G (1963) Compensatory adaptation of renal function in the unanaesthetized rat. Am J Physiol 205:1042–1048

Peters G (1979) History and problems of compensatory adaptation of renal functions and of compensatory hypertrophy in the kidney. In: Peters G, Diezi J, Guignard J-P (eds) Renal adaptation to nephron loss. Karger, Basel, pp 1–11

Potter DE, Leumann EP, Sakai T, Holliday MA (1972) Early response of glomerular filtration rate to unilateral nephrectomy. Kidney Int 5:131–136

Provoost AP, Molenaar JC (1980a) Changes in glomerular filtration rate after unilateral nephrectomy in rats. Pflugers Arch 385:161–165

Provoost AP, Molenaar JC (1980b) Nierenfunktion während und nach einseitiger Ureterobstruktion bei der Ratte. Urologe A 19:8–10

Provoost AP, Molenaar JC (1981) Renal function during and after a temporary complete unilateral ureter obstruction in rats. Invest Urol 18:242–246

Provoost AP, de Keijzer MH, Kort WJ, Wolff ED, Molenaar JC (1982) The glomerular filtration rate of isogeneically transplanted rat kidneys. Kidney Int 21:459–465

Provoost AP, de Keijzer MH, Wolff ED, Molenaar JC (1983) Development of renal function in the rat. The measurement of GFR and ERPF and correlation to body and kidney weight. Renal Physiol 6:1–9

Provoost AP, de Keijzer MH, Kort WJ, van Aken M, Weyma IM, Wolff ED, Molenaar JC (1984a) The influence of the recipient upon renal function after isogeneic kidney transplantation in the rat. Transplantation 37:55–62

Provoost AP, Wolff Ed, de Keijzer MH, Molenaar JC (1984b) Influence of the recipient's size upon renal function following kidney transplantation. An experimental and clinical investigation. J Pediatr Surg 19:63–67

Purkerson ML, Hoffsten PE, Klahr S (1976) Pathogenesis of the glomerulopathy associated with renal infarction in rats. Kidney Int 9:407–417

Purkerson ML, Joist JH, Greenberg JM, Kay D, Hoffstein PE, Klahr S (1982) Inhibition by anticoagulant drugs of the progressive hypertension and uremia associated with renal infarction in rats. Thromb Res 26:227–240

Robitaille P, Mongeau J-G, Lortie L, Sinnassamy P (1985) Long-term follow-up of patients who underwent unilateral nephrectomy in childhood. Lancet i:1297–1299

Rowe JW, Andres R, Tobin JD, Norris AH, Shock NW (1976) The effect of age on creatinine clearance in men: a cross-sectional and longitudinal study. J Gerontol 31:155–163

Salusky I, Kleinknecht C, Broyer M, Gubler M-C (1981) Prolonged renal survival and stunting, with protein-deficient diets in experimental uremia. J Lab Clin Med 97:21–30

Sands J, Dobbing J, Gratrix CA (1979) Cell number and cell size: organ growth and development and the control of catch-up growth in rats. Lancet ii:503–505

Seyer-Hansen K, Gundersen HJG, Osterby R (1985) Stereology of the rat kidney during compensatory renal hypertrophy. Acta Pathol Microbiol Immunol Scand [A] 93:9–12

Shimamura T, Morrison AB (1975) A progressive glomerulosclerosis occurring in partial five-sixths nephrectomized rats. Am J Pathol 79:95–101

Shirley DG, Skinner J (1978) Acute compensatory adaptation of renal function following contralateral kidney exclusion in Brattleboro rats with diabetes insipidus. J Physiol (Lond) 283:425–438

Simon J, Zamora I, Mendizabal S, Castel V, Lurbe A (1982) Glomerulotubular balance and functional compensation in nephrectomized children. Nephron 31:203–208

Smith S, Laprad P, Grantham J (1985) Long-term effect of uninephrectomy on serum creatinine concentration and arterial blood pressure. Am J Kidn Dis 6:143–148

Sterioff S (1985) Unilateral nephrectomy in living related kidney donors is safe and beneficial. Mayo Clin Proc 60:423–424

Striker GE, Nagle RB, Kohnen PW, Smuckler EA (1969) Response to unilateral nephrectomy in old rats. Arch Pathol 87:439–442

Sutherland DER (1985) Living related donors should be used whenever possible. Transplant Proc 17:1503–1509

Thorner PS, Arbus GS, Celeremajer DS, Baumal R (1984) Focal segmental glomerulosclerosis and progressive renal failure associated with a unilateral kidney. Pediatrics 73:806–810

Tsuruda H, Okuda S, Onoyama K, Oh Y, Fujishima M (1986) Effect of blood pressure on the progress of renal deterioration in rats with renal mass reduction. J Lab Clin Med 107:43–50

Tucker BJ, Blantz RC (1977) An analysis of the determinants of nephron filtration rate. Am J Physiol 232:F477–F483

Vincenti F, Amend WJC, Kaysen G, Feduska N, Birnbaum J, Duca R, Salvatierra O (1983) Long-term renal function in kidney donors. Transplantation 36:626–629

Weiland D, Sutherland DER, Chavers B, Simmons RL, Ascher NL, Najarian JS (1984) Information on 628 living related kidney donors at a single institution, with long-term follow-up in 472 cases. Transplant Proc 16:5–7

Winick M, Noble A (1965) Quantitative changes in DNA, RNA and protein during prenatal and postnatal growth in the rat. Dev Biol 12:451–466

Zuchelli P, Cagnoli L, Casanova S, Donini U, Pasquali S (1983) Focal glomerulosclerosis in patients with unilateral nephrectomy. Kidney Int 24:649–655

Urological Operations for Solitary Kidneys in Children

F.-J. Helmig, D. Vogl, and K. Devens

Summary

Depending on the underlying disease, children with solitary kidneys who have to undergo urological operations have the same good or poor prognosis as children with two kidneys (Whiting et al. 1983; Redman and Birsada 1976; Stackl et al. 1983). However, the problem of long-term prognosis persists. It is similar to that for children who have undergone surgery for reflux: a certain number of them will develop renal insufficiency in 20–30 years. Nephrologists estimate that 20% of adults who suffer from renal insufficiency and become dialysis dependent formerly had reflux nephropathy. The influence of reimplantation, performed with good results during the past few years, cannot be assessed so far. Large prospective studies are needed.

Zusammenfassung

Wenn Kinder mit Solitärnieren urologisch operiert werden müssen, haben sie, je nach Befund und Art der Grunderkrankung, die gleich gute oder schlechte Prognose wie Kinder mit zwei Organen (Whiting et al. 1983; Redman and Birsada 1976; Stackl et al. 1983). Damit bleibt jedoch das Problem der Langzeitprognose bestehen. Es ist das gleiche wie bei allen Kindern, die wegen Reflux operiert worden sind und bei denen man, statistisch gesehen, rechnen muß, daß eine Anzahl von ihnen in 20 bis 30 Jahren niereninsuffizient werden wird. Nephrologen rechnen damit, daß etwa 20% der Erwachsenen, die niereninsuffizient und dialyseabhängig werden, ursprünglich eine Refluxnephropathie hatten. Über die Beeinflussung dieses Verlaufs durch die in den letzten Jahren mit gutem Erfolg durchgeführte Reimplantation läßt sich zum heutigen Zeitpunkt noch nichts aussagen. Dazu bedarf es größerer prospektiver Studien.

Résumé

Selon l'affection sous-jacente, les enfants n'ayant qu'un seul rein et devant subir une intervention urologique ont un pronostic ne présentant aucune différence significative par rapport aux enfants normaux (Whiting et al. 1983; Redman et Bir-

---

Pediatric Surgical Clinic, Dr. von Hauner'sches Kinderspital of the University of Munich, Lindwurmstr. 4, D-8000 Munich 2, Federal Republic of Germany

Progress in Pediatric Surgery, Vol. 23
Ed. by L. Spitz et al.
© Springer-Verlag Berlin Heidelberg 1989

sada 1976; Stackl et al. 1983). Toutefois le problème du pronostic à long terme demeure. Il s'agit du même problème que celui posé par les enfants opérés pour reflux. Dans le cas de ces enfants, il faut s'attendre statistiquement à ce qu'un certain nombre d'entre eux présenteront une insuffisance néphrétique après 20 à 30 ans. Les néphrologues estiment que 20% environ des adultes présentant une insuffisance néphrétique et devant être dialysés auraient présenté initialement une néphropathie de reflux. Il est encore trop tôt pour prévoir une évolution à long terme malgré une technique de réimplantation utilisée depuis quelques années avec succès. Il faudra attendre les résultats d'études prospectives à grande échelle.

Introduction

In the treatment of urologically diseased solitary kidneys, the indications for surgery and the prognosis are the same as those for patients with two kidneys.

Patients

From 1970 to 1983, 33 children with solitary kidneys underwent urological operations at the Pediatric Surgical Clinic of Dr. von Haunersches Kinderspital of the

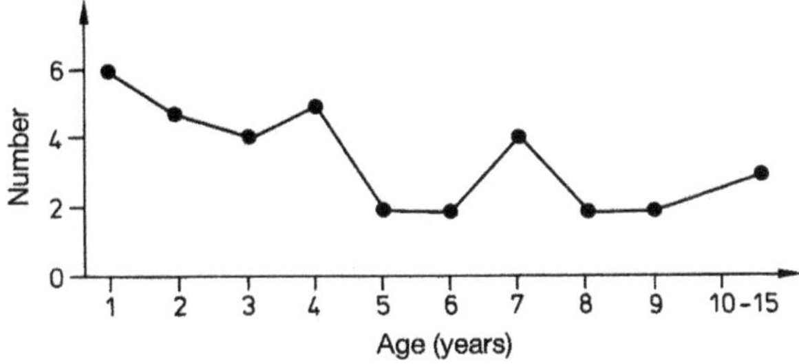

Fig. 1. Age distribution of children with solitary kidney

Table 1. Causes of solitary kidney in 33 children

Agenesis	7	
Nephrectomy	26	
For – pyelonephritic renal shrinkage		15
– tumour		2
– calculi		1
– hydronephrosis		4
– renal cysts		1
– multiple malformations		3
Preceeding operations:		
– reimplantation		4
– pole resection		3
– ureterostomy		2
– transurethral valve resection		1

F.-J. Helmig et al.

Table 2. Urological operations performed in 33 children with solitary kidneys

Reimplantation	17
Tumour excision	2
Lithotomy	2
Pyeloplasty	5
Ureterostomy	3
Ileal conduit	1
Transurethral valve resection	3

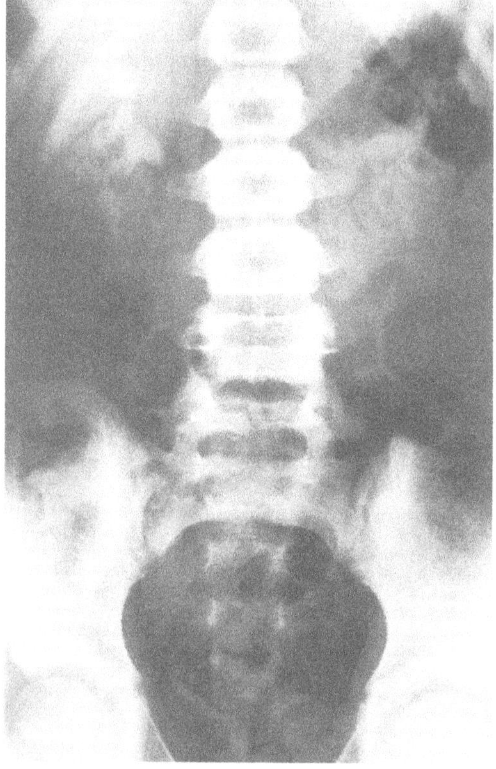

Fig. 2. An 8-year-old girl with nephrectomy on the left side and pyelic calculi in the remaining solitary kidney

University of Munich. There were 16 boys and 17 girls. Solitary kidneys were located on the right side in 21 instances and on the left side in 12 instances. The age distribution is shown in Fig. 1.

The causes of solitary kidney in our 33 cases are listed in Table 1. Pyelonephritic renal shrinkage includes cases that developed following myelomeningocele or posterior urethral valves. The tumours mentioned were both Wilms' tumours.

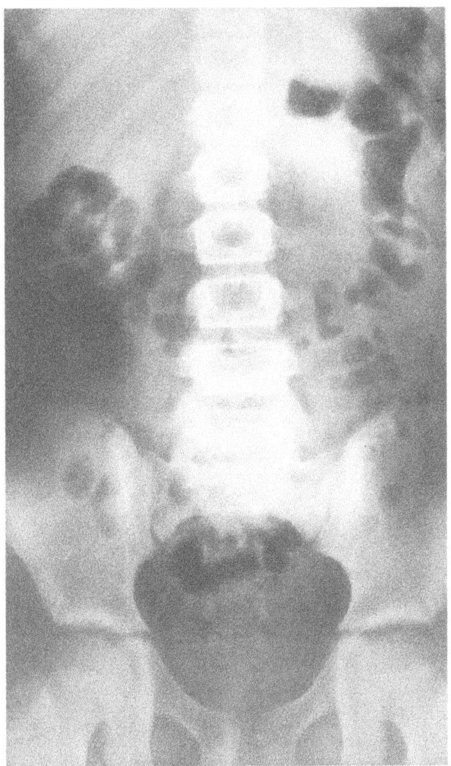

Fig. 3. Same patient as in Fig. 2 after pyelolithotomy

Multiple malformations consisted, for instance, in a combination of pelvic kidney
with reflux or with anorectal atresia.

Operations

Operations that were performed in these children with solitary kidneys are listed
in Table 2. Notably, three transurethral valve resections are mentioned; this is
due to the fact that nephrectomies had been performed in these children elsewhere and the residual urethral valves were resected later.

Only two of our patients developed renal insufficiency, one of whom had un-
recognized posterior urethral valves. Since nephrectomy had already been carried
out elsewhere, we had first to do a transurethral valve resection and then to establish a ureterostomy due to the impaired function of the solitary kidney. In spite of
this, renal insufficiency with hypertonus developed and the patient is presently
dialysis dependent.

The other patient with renal insufficiency had been nephrectomized elsewhere
at the age of 6 years for silent kidney due to pyelic calculi and empyema. Two

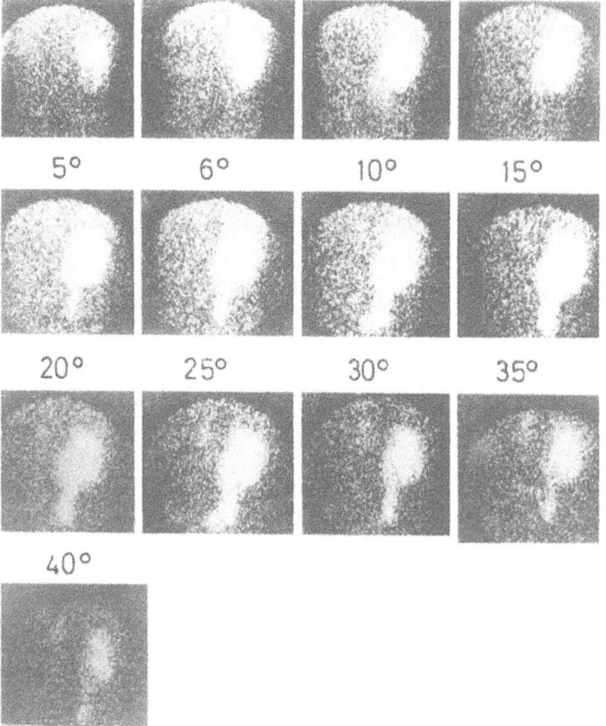

Fig. 4. Scintiscan in a 2-year-old boy with posterior urethral valves and bilateral distal ureteral stenosis: nearly functionless kidney on the left side and impaired urinary drainage on the right

years later, she was referred to us for treatment of pyelic calculi of the other kidney (Fig. 2). Since a nephrotomy was too dangerous in the solitary kidney, we performed a pyelotomy to remove the accessible calculi, mainly from the pelvis and the intermediate calices. Since intraoperative sonographical localization of renal calculi was not possible 10 years ago, residual calculi which did not impair urinary drainage had to be left in place (Fig. 3).

The underlying disease was diagnosed only after this operation: tubular acidosis and nephrocalcinosis, untreatable by alkalisation in this stage. Seven years after the last operation, the patient is awaiting dialysis and transplantation for progressive renal insufficiency.

There was a satisfactory postoperative course in all other patients, regarding both renal function and the prophylaxis and treatment of infections.

Two cases are presented as examples:

1. A 2-year-old boy with posterior urethral valves and bilateral, distal ureteral stenosis was nephrectomized on the left side, since qualitative iodine-hippuric acid clearance revealed a residual function of only 5%. A ureterostomy was established on the right side. A preoperative scintiscan revealed a nearly functionless

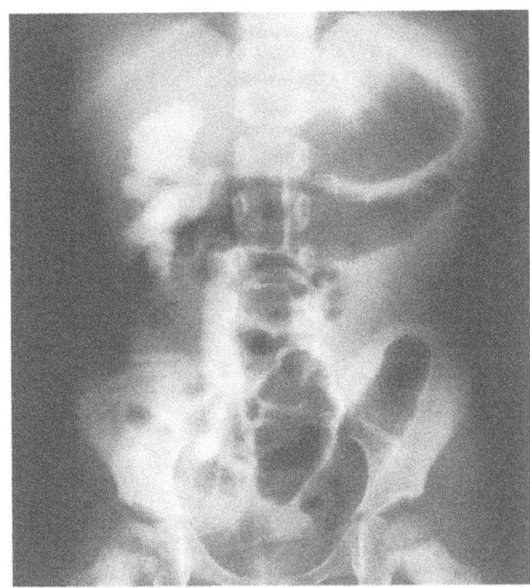

Fig. 5. Intravenous pyelogram in the same patient as in Fig. 4 at the time of transurethral valve resection and establishment of ureterostomy

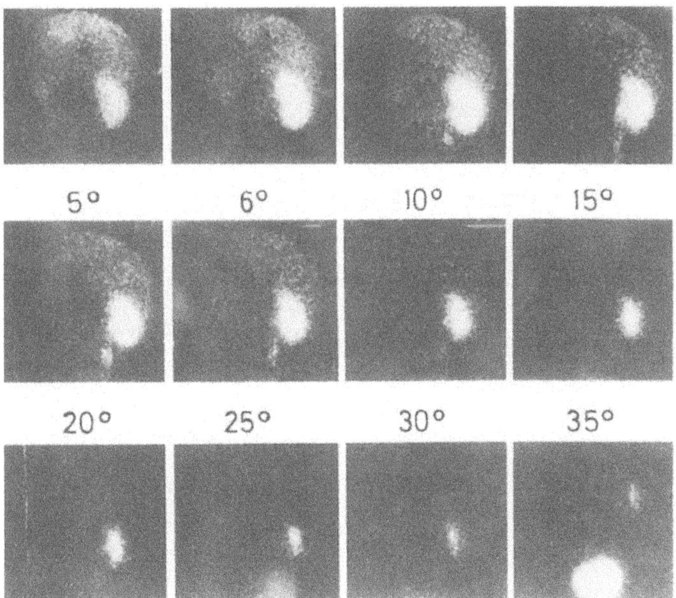

Fig. 6. Scintiscan of the same patient 1 year following reimplantation of the right ureter reveals good urinary drainage

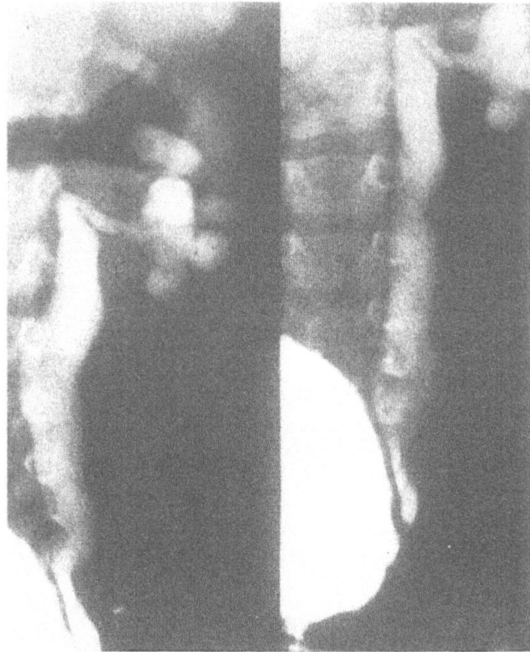

Fig. 7. Micturition cystourethrogram of a 3-year-old boy with right-sided renal agenesis and distal ureteral stenosis with VUR on the left side

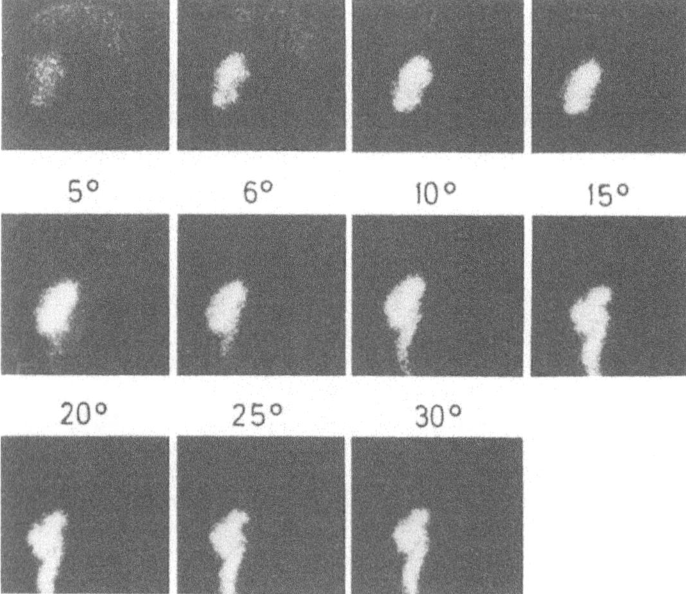

Fig. 8. Scintiscan in the same patient as in Fig. 7 prior to surgery shows grossly delayed urinary drainage

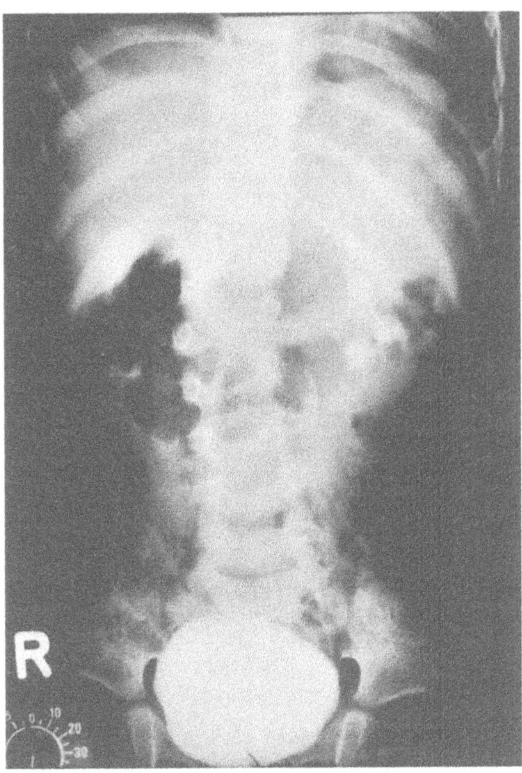

Fig. 9. Intravenous pyelogram of the same patient following reimplantation of the left ureter

kidney on the left side as well as impaired urinary drainage on the right (Fig. 4). Figure 5 shows the right kidney at the time of transurethral valve resection and establishment of a ureterostomy. One year later, the right ureter was reimplanted. A control scintiscan, again 1 year later, shows good urinary drainage on the right side (Fig. 6).

2. A 3-year-old boy was referred for treatment of right-sided renal agenesis and distal ureteral stenosis with VUR on the left (Figs. 7 and 8). The left ureter was reimplanted using Leadbetter and Politano's method; this achieved good urinary drainage (Fig. 9). Maintenance of good urinary drainage was confirmed by scintiscan 2 years after the operation (Fig. 10).

One of the two Wilms' tumors in solitary kidneys was sparingly excised and the other enucleated. The children are free of recurrence 4 and 5 years respectively following surgery. In one of them a pole resection was performed; in the other, frozen sections revealed a diffuse infiltration of the whole kidney (nephroblastomatosis). Following irradiation and adjuvant chemotherapy, a second-look operation revealed no residual tumor tissue. In this context, the papers by Morales et al. (1981), Brannen et al. (1983) and Schiff et al. (1979) should be referred to.

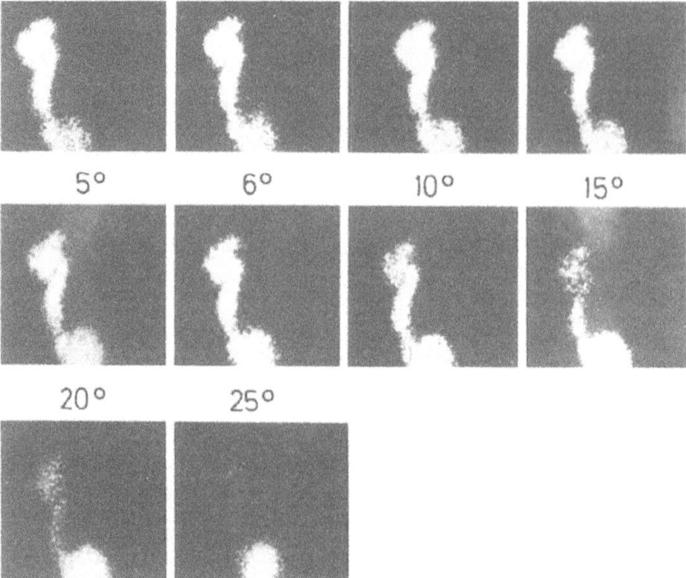

Fig. 10. Scintiscan shows maintenance of good urinary drainage in same patient 2 years after operation

Iodine-hippuric acid clearance revealed renal function at the lower border of the age-corresponding norm in all of our patients with solitary kidney, but without signs of deterioration or increased urea or creatinine (Heinz 1967; Costantini et al. 1969).

There was no question of saving the diseased organ in the children who developed renal insufficiency, and it would have made no difference in the incurable underlying disease.

References

1. Brannen GE, Correa RJ, Gibbons RP (1983) Renal cell carcinoma in solitary kidneys. J Urol 129:130–131
2. Costantini A, Sodi A, Durval A, et al (1969) Physiopathologie der Einzelniere. Urologe 8: 37–38
3. Heinz J (1967) Das Lebensschicksal der Einnierigen. Verlag Volk und Gesundheit, Berlin
4. Morales L, Rovira J, Mongard M, et al (1981) Solitary pelvic kidney and neuroblastoma in a child. J Urol 126:249–250
5. Redman JF, Birsada NK (1976) Extensive nephrolithotomy in previously operated solitary kidneys. J Urol 115:502–504
6. Schiff M Jr, Bagley DH, Lytton B (1979) Treatment of solitary and bilateral renal carcinomas. J Urol 121:581–583
7. Stackl W, Hofmann E, Marberger, et al (1983) Is the solitary kidney a privileged kidney? Br J Urol 55:460–464
8. Whiting JC, Stanisic TH, Drach EW, et al (1983) Congenital ureteral valves: report of 2 patients including one with a solitary kidney and associated hypertension. J Urol 129:1222–1226

Reconstructive Surgery in Eight Children with Solitary Kidneys

O. H. Nielsen and J. Thorup

Summary

Within a 10-year period reconstructive urinary tract surgery has been carried out in eight children with solitary kidneys. The children were 0–5 years old. Six had unilateral renal agenesis and two had unilateral multicystic kidney. In five children ureteroneocystostomy was performed, in two of them because of reflux. In two children pyeloureteroplasty was performed, and in one both ureteroneocystostomy and pyeloureteroplasty. The multicystic kidneys were removed.

The renal function was poor preoperatively in five children; two of these also had urosepsis. These children were all under 15 months of age. Postoperatively, the renal function was subnormal (although improved) in two children; in six it was normal.

The most important prognostic factors in solitary kidneys with urinary tract obstruction are infection and developmental injury.

Zusammenfassung

In einer zehnjährigen Periode sind bei acht einnierigen Patienten rekonstruktive Harnwegsoperationen ausgeführt worden. Die Kinder waren 0–5 Jahre alt. Sechs hatten unilaterale Nierenagenesie, zwei hatten unilaterale multicystische Niere. Bei fünf Kindern wurde Ureteroneocystostomie durchgeführt wegen Striktur (3) oder Reflux (2). Zwei Kinder unterzogen sich einer Pyeloplastik und eines sowohl einer Ureteroneocystostomie als auch einer Pyeloplastik. Die multicystischen Nieren wurden entfernt.

Die Nierenfunktion war präoperativ in fünf Fällen schlecht; zwei von diesen Kindern hatten dazu Urosepsis. Diese Kinder waren alle unter 15 Monate alt.

Postoperativ war die Nierenfunktion bei zwei Kindern subnormal (aber verbessert), bei sechs Kindern normal.

Die wichtigsten prognostischen Faktoren bei Einzelnieren mit Harnwegsobstruktion sind Infektion und pränatale Beschädigung.

Résumé

En l'espace de dix ans, il a été procédé dans le cas de huit patients avec un rein unique, à des opérations des voies urinaires à des fins de reconstruction. Les en-

University Clinic of Paediatric Surgery, Rigshospitalet, DK-2100 Copenhagen Ø, Denmark

Progress in Pediatric Surgery, Vol. 23
Ed. by L. Spitz et al.
© Springer-Verlag Berlin Heidelberg 1989

fants étaient âgés de 0 à 5 ans. Six d'entre eux présentaient une agénésie rénale unilatérale, deux d'entre eux un rein unilatéral multicystique. Dans le cas de cinq enfants, il fut procédé à une urétéro-néocystostomie pour reflux. Dans deux cas on pratiqua una urétéro-plastie pour stricture ou reflux. Deux enfants subirent une pyéloplastie et dans un cas on pratiqua une urétéro-néocystostomie et une pyélourétéroplastie. On pratiqua une néphrectomie pour les deux multicystiques.

La fonction rénale était insuffisante dans le cas de cinq enfants avant l'intervention. Deux d'entre eux présentaient aussi une infection urinaire. Ces enfants avaient tous moins de 15 mois. Après l'intervention, la fonction rénale était subnormale (mais améliorée) dans deux cas et normale dans six cas.

Les facteurs pronostiques d'une importance majeure dans les cas de rein unique avec obstruction des voies rénales sont l'infection et les lésions causées par des embryopathies.

Correct management of obstructive uropathy is particularly important in children with a solitary kidney. Fortunately, congenital solitary kidney with outflow obstruction is a rare condition. Although, from a functional point of view, many children with bilateral or infravesical obstruction are in the same situation, we have chosen to report only cases with contralateral renal agenesis or multicystic kidney.

Material and Methods

At the Department of Paediatric Surgery, Rigshospitalet, University of Copenhagen, in the 10-year period from 1975 to 1984 we saw 16 children with unilateral renal agenesis. Ten of these cases were diagnosed incidentally, often in the course of routine investigation for anal atresia or other anomalies. The remaining six cases were diagnosed based on symptoms from the obstructed solitary kidney.

During the same period, 15 children with a unilateral multicystic kidney were seen. Two of them had contralateral obstruction.

The diagnostic investigations were ultrasonic scanning, intravenous pyelography and renal scintiscan. Renal function was evaluated with renography and creatinine clearance preoperatively and during follow-up. The age of the patients at the time of diagnosis was 0–5 years. Their clinical data are listed in Table 1.

A primary reconstruction was the routine method, but in two cases temporary urinary deviation was indicated due to infection or because immediate surgery could not be undertaken. In one boy with bladder dysfunction recurrence of vesicoureteral reflux indicated reoperation.

Results

There were no deaths or serious complications. The outflow obstruction was eliminated in all cases.

Table 1. Clinical data of eight children with urinary tract obstruction and solitary kidney

Case no.	Age at diagnosis	Presenting symptoms	Diagnosis	Operative procedures
1	Prenatal	Prenatal ultra-sonography	Left multicystic kidney Right pyeloureteral and ureterovesical obstruction	Left nephrectomy Right ureteroneocystostomy Temporary right nephrostomy (percutaneous) Right pyeloureteroplasty (Anderson-Hynes)
2	3 weeks	Adrenogenital syndrome	Left multicystic kidney Right pyeloureteral obstruction	Left nephrectomy Right pyeloureteroplasty (Anderson-Hynes)
3	3 weeks	Uraemia	Left renal agenesis Right ureterovesical obstruction	Right ureteroneocystostomy
4	8 months	Urosepsis	Left renal agenesis Right megaureter with vesicoureteral reflux	Right ureteroneocystostomy with tapering of the ureter
5	10 months	Urinary tract infection, lower abdominal mass	Right renal agenesis Left megaureter with ureterovesical obstruction Hydrometrocolpos	Left ureteroneocystostomy Incision of vaginal septum
6	15 months	Urosepsis	Left renal agenesis Right megaureter with ureterovesical obstruction	Temporary right ureterostomy Right ureteroneocystostomy Closure of ureterocutaneous fistula
7	4 years	Urinary tract infection	Left renal agenesis Right vesicoureteral reflux Neurogenic bladder Occult spina bifida	Right ureteroneocystostomy Reoperation 1 year later
8	5 years	Post-traumatic haematuria	Right renal agenesis Left pyeloureteral obstruction	Left pyeloureteroplasty (Anderson-Hynes)

Five children had severe deterioration of renal function at the time of diagnosis (creatinine clearance below 50% of the normal value for the age). These children were all under 15 months of age, and two of them also had sepsis.

In three cases renal function was normalised after surgery. In the remaining two cases it was improved, but still subnormal. These children were both neonates, and both had severe obstruction. They were operated at the ages of 12 and 19 days. None of them developed infection.

Discussion

The presence of a solitary kidney is often the result of a developmental error, and it is not surprising that the frequency of obstructive anomalies is high. Because of the potential threat to renal function, the obstruction assumes an importance equal to that of bilateral or infravesical obstruction in patients with two kidneys. Our experience with this small group of patients confirms that normal renal function may result from the relief of urinary tract obstruction connected with a solitary kidney. In two of our cases there was a probably permanent decrease in renal function. In both cases the decrease existed preoperatively, and in fact was present at the time of birth. It is possible, and seems probable, that the functional injury had already occurred during the early fetal development of the kidney (Beck 1971).

Reference

Beck AD (1971) The effect of intrauterine urinary obstruction upon the development of the fetal kidney. J Urol 105:784–789

Surgery on Solitary Kidneys in Childhood

H.-D. Jaeger and G. Gutsche

Summary

From 1969 to 1984, 31 children were operated on for a diseased solitary kidney. There was a peak of incidence during the first 2 years of life, due mostly to congenitally malformed solitary kidneys. In contrast, operations in older children became necessary for diseased residual kidneys. In some children, secondary or even multiple operations had to be performed in order to maintain satisfactory organ function. Except in three preuraemic patients, renal functions were fully compensatory during a follow-up of 1–16 years. Former reservations regarding surgical intervention in solitary kidneys should be dropped in the face of these good operative results.

Zusammenfassung

Zwischen 1969 und 1985 wurden 31 Kinder wegen Erkrankungen einer Solitärniere operiert. Ein Häufigkeitsgipfel fand sich in den beiden ersten Lebensjahren, überwiegend an kongenitalen fehlgebildeten Einzelnieren. Dagegen waren die Eingriffe bei älteren Kindern in der Regel wegen erkrankter Restnieren notwendig. Bei einigen Patienten machten sich Sekundär- oder gar Mehrfachoperationen erforderlich, um eine befriedigende Restfunktion des Organs zu erhalten. Während einer Nachbeobachtungszeit von 1–16 Jahren bewegten sich die Nierenleistungen im Bereich der vollen Kompensation, bis auf drei prä-urämische Patienten. Die früher geübte Zurückhaltung gegenüber operativen Interventionen an Einzelnieren muß unter dem Eindruck der überwiegend guten Behandlungsergebnisse fallengelassen werden.

Résumé

Entre 1969 et 1984, 31 enfants ont été opérés pour une affection d'un rein unique. L'intervention a été le plus souvent pratiquée durant les deux premières années de vie et était due à des malformations congénitales du rein unique. Dans le cas des enfants plus âgés par contre, l'intervention était due, en règle générale, à une affection du rein résiduel. Dans le cas de certains patients, il fallut pratiquer soit

Paediatric Surgical Clinic, Karl Marx University of Leipzig, Oststr. 21, 7050 Leipzig, German Democratic Republic

Progress in Pediatric Surgery, Vol. 23
Ed. by L. Spitz et al.
© Springer-Verlag Berlin Heidelberg 1989

une intervention secondaire soit même des interventions multiples pour pouvoir conserver une fonction rénale résiduelle suffisante. Ces patients ont été suivis de 1 à 16 ans et la fonction rénale était proche de la compensation totale, à l'exception de trois patients pré-urémiques. Ces résultats étant donc satisfaisants en majorité, il n'y a plus lieu d'hésiter à intervenir chirurgicalement sur un rein unique, comme cela se faisait souvent autrefois.

Solitary kidneys are the result of either renal agenesis/aplasia or nephrectomy of the contralateral organ. Functional solitary kidneys due to disease of the other kidney will not be discussed here. Although a solitary kidney is able to adapt by virtue of compensatory hypertrophy, it reaches only about two thirds of the functional maximum of two healthy organs. Thus, compensatory renal capacity is clearly limited, carrying the danger of an acute renal insufficiency in case of disease or surgical insult to the solitary organ.

Recently, Stackl et al. (1983) disproved in animal experiments the assumption that a hypertrophied solitary kidney is more resistant to insults such as colibacillosis or ischaemic damage. The extent to which these findings are transferrable to the human being remains open. According to Dees (1960), solitary kidneys are actually more prone to complications. He found late complications in 66% of congenital solitary kidneys as compared with 37% of acquired solitary kidneys. In the face of these pathophysiological relations, the indication for diagnosis and therapy assumes an extraordinary importance. As far as we know, no large studies concerning this topic have been published in the paediatric surgical and paediatric urological literature.

We report on 31 patients with solitary kidneys who have undergone surgery of the upper urinary tract at our clinic since 1969. As far as age distribution is con-

Table 1. Underlying disease leading to decreased kidney function and finally nephrectomy

Condition	No. of cases
Stenosis of the ureteropelvic junction	3
Ostial stenosis	2
Vesicoureteral reflux	6
Urethral stenosis	5
Cysts	1
Megaureter syndrome	1
Ureterocele	1
Neurogenic bladder	1
Bladder exstrophy	1
	$n = 21$

Table 2. Operations performed on solitary kidneys

Operation	No.
Heminephrectomy	1
Pyeloplasty	4
Ureterolysis	6
Ureterocystostomy	8
Antireflux plasty	12
Ureterosigmoidostomy	2
Cutaneous ureterostomy	5
Others	14
	$n = 52$

Table 3. Indications for primary intervention in solitary and residual kidneys

	Solitary kidney	Residual kidney
Stenosis of the ureteropelvic junction	–	6
Ureteral stenosis	3	2
Ostial stenosis	1	2
Vesicoureteral reflux	5	9
Other stenosis	–	2
Wilms' tumour	1	–
	$n = 10$	$n = 21$

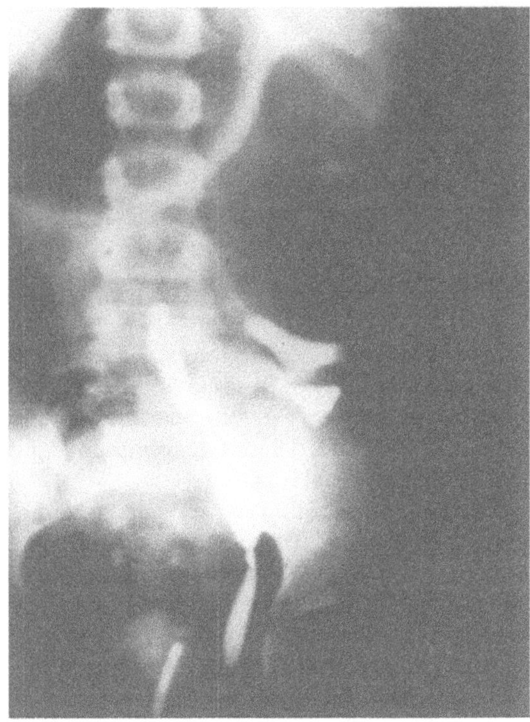

Fig. 1. Wilms' tumour in a left-sided solitary kidney

cerned, there was a preponderance of interventions during the first 2 years of life, whereby operations for congenital solitary kidney slightly predominated, whereas operations on residual kidneys became necessary chiefly in older children. Ten children had congenital solitary kidneys, 21 residual kidneys. Causes of renal loss are listed in Table 1.

A total of 52 operations had to be carried out in the 31 children with solitary kidneys. Temporary urinary diversions and definitive operations can be distin-

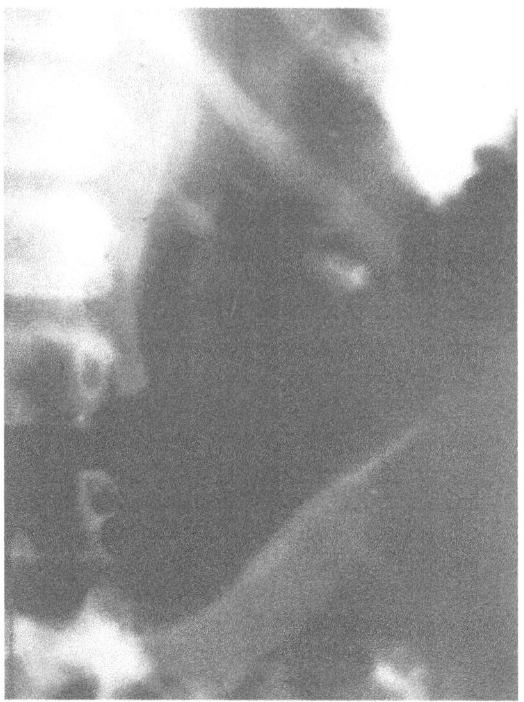

Fig. 2. Follow-up urogram 2 years after tumour excision in the same patient

guished. The types of operations are shown in Table 2, the indications for primary intervention in Table 3. In some of the children secondary or even multiple operations became necessary. Seven operations of the upper urinary tract had to be carried out in one child. These interventions required great surgical skill to conserve even borderline renal function.

Except for one child with a Wilms' tumour, our patients had exclusively congenital malformations combined with disturbances of urinary transport. Emergency situations must be given special attention, since they require immediate decisions. For instance, a Wilms' tumour had to be excised from the upper pole of a left-sided solitary kidney in a 3-year-old boy (Fig. 1). An i.v. pyelogram following tumour excision showed sufficient function of the residual organ (Fig. 2).

Surprisingly, there was no nephrolithiasis of a solitary kidney among our patients, although this is reported rather frequently in the literature. We were also fortunate not to have to treat primary or secondary purulent suppurating pyelonephritis or tuberculous inflammations.

Follow-up in our patients ranged from 1 to 16 years, with an average of 7.5 years. With the exception of three children, the serum creatinine levels of our patients are within the compensatory range.

Most of the children show normal growth pre- as well as postoperatively, with one girl even exhibiting accelerated growth. Only one boy shows retarded growth and one girl dwarfism, both children having preuraemic serum creatinine levels.

In the future, prenatal ultrasonography will contribute to the early diagnosis of solitary kidneys and allow early surgical intervention to protect and improve organ function. The view that one should hesitate to intervene surgically in solitary kidneys can no longer be defended in the face of these predominantly positive results.

References

Dees JE (1960) Prognosis of the solitary kidney. J Urol 85:550–552
Emanuel B, Nachman R, Aronson N, Weiss H (1974) Congenital solitary kidney. Am J Dis Child 127:17–19
Rockstroh H (1967) Das Lebensschicksal der Einnierigen. Berlin, VEB Volk und Gesundheit
Stackl W, Hofmann E, Marberger M (1983) Solitary kidney a privileged kidney. Br J Urol 55: 460–464

Outcome Following Surgery
for Solitary Kidney in Children

K. Gdanietz and G. Piehl

Summary

We reviewed 8700 urological patients treated as inpatients over a period of 30 years, among them 386 children with primary or secondary solitary kidneys. Forty-one of these children had to undergo surgery for secondary pathological conditions of their solitary kidney. Diagnosis, treatment and results are analysed and tabulated for 20 primary and 21 secondary solitary kidneys.

Generally, the prognosis of a primary solitary kidney is poorer than that of a secondary solitary kidney. Patients who have to undergo dialysis belong to the group with primary solitary kidneys. The worst prognosis is that for the combination of subvesical stenosis and associated uropathy.

Zusammenfassung

Es wird eine Übersichtsarbeit über ein Krankengut von 30 Jahren mit 8700 stationär behandelten urologischen Patienten, das 386 Kinder mit einer primären beziehungsweise sekundären Einzelniere enthält, gegeben. 41 dieser Kinder mußten wegen Sekundärpathologien an ihrer Einzelniere operiert werden. Analysiert und tabellarisch zusammengefaßt werden Diagnose, Therapie and Ergebnis von 20 primären und 21 sekundären Einzelnieren.

Das Schicksal von Kindern mit einer primären Einzelniere verläuft insgesamt ungünstiger als das von Kindern mit einer sekundären Einzelniere. Patienten, die in das Dialyseprogramm aufgenommen werden mußten, rekrutieren sich aus der Gruppe der primären Einzelnieren. Von allen Diagnosen ist die Kombination subvesikale Obstruktion und assoziierte Uropathie die problematischte Konstellation.

Résumé

Il s'agit d'une étude rétrospective s'étendant sur une période de 30 ans et traitant de 8700 cas de patients hospitalisés pour traitement urologique, dont 386 enfants avec un rein unique primaire ou secondaire. 41 de ces enfants ont subi une intervention pour évolution pathologique de leur rein unique. Nous avons groupé dans

Paediatric Surgical Clinic, Klinikum Berlin-Buch, Karower Str. 11, 1115 Berlin-Buch, German Democratic Republic

Progress in Pediatric Surgery, Vol. 23
Ed. by L. Spitz et al.
© Springer-Verlag Berlin Heidelberg 1989

un tableau les données obtenues concernant le diagnostic, la thérapeutique et les résultats dans le cas de 20 reins uniques primaires et de 21 reins uniques secondaires. Nous avons constaté que l'évolution est moins favorable dans le cas des enfants présentant un rein unique primaire que dans le cas de ceux ayant un rein unique secondaire. Les patients qui ont dû être intégrés au programme de dialyse avaient tous un rein unique primaire. Le pronostic le plus réservé est celui qui correspond à une sténose vésicale avec uropathie associée.

Introduction

A review of the fate of children who had to undergo surgery of solitary kidneys over a period of 30 years requires a perception of former therapeutic methods applied according to the state of art at the time in question.

After 30 years' experience in the field of pediatric urology we are aware of the fact that we would proceed today differently than we did years ago. The collaboration of various disciplines and the development of new techniques have improved diagnosis, thus rendering earlier treatment possible.

As far as our review is concerned, we must state that only casuistic reports could disclose the fate of our patients in detail, since the problems are not always limited to the kidney. Combined malformations increase the problems.

Since detailed casuistic reports are beyond the scope of this paper, we present our patient series summarized according to the diagnosis of primary and secondary solitary kidneys. Only two cases with rare diagnoses are described in some detail.

Patients

Among 8700 urological inpatients treated from 1956 to 1985 (maldescended testicles, hydroceles, varicoceles and tumours not included) were 386 children with solitary kidneys. Only 41 of these children, however, had to undergo surgery of the solitary kidney. In the remaining children solitary kidneys were found along with anorectal malformations or incidentally in diseases of other origin, or were the result of nephrectomies.

We distinguish between congenital, i.e. primary, and acquired, i.e. secondary, solitary kidneys.

Primary Solitary Kidneys ($n = 20$)

The indications for surgical intervention are summarized in Table 1 under the column headed "Diagnoses". Problems arose in all of the children. Because of their rareness, two diseases are described in some detail.

Table 1. Diagnoses, treatment and assessment in surgical interventions of primary solitary kidneys

	Sex	Stenosis of ureteropelvic junction	Vesicoureteral reflux	Ostial stenosis	Ureteral dystopia	Retrocaval ureter	Gartner cysts	Nephrolithiasis	Trauma	Age at onset of disease (years)	Age at initiation of treatment (years)	Age at initiation of surgical treatment (years)	Therapy	No. of operations	Assessment[a]	Age at follow-up (years)	Length of follow-up (years)	Remarks
1	m	X								$6/12$	$6/12$	$6/12$	Anderson-Hynes pyeloplasty	1	2	11	11	
2	m	X								1	2	2	Anderson-Hynes pyeloplasty	2	2	15	13	
3	f	X								$1/12$	$1/12$	1	Nephrostomy	1	2	16	16	Bladder exstrophy, anal atresia
4	f	X								$2/12$	$2/12$	$5/12$	Anderson-Hynes pyeloplasty	1	2	8	8	
5	m	X									13	14	Nephrostomy	1	†			Died elsewhere
6	f	Y	X							1	1	2	ARP, Anderson-Hynes pyeloplasty, revision, T-drainage	3	1	7	5	
7	m		X							5	5	7	ARP, UCN, ARP	3	2	16	9	
8	m		X							$1/12$	$1/12$	9	ARP	1	3	11	11	
9	f			X						3	3	3	UCN	1	1	10	7	

No.	Sex												Procedure					Remarks
10	m			X				Y		5/12	5/12	5/12	Cutaneous ureterostomy, UCN	2	3	14	14	Anal atresia
11	m			X				Y		7	7	9	Lower pole resection, UCN, cutaneous ureterostomy, UCN	5	4	25	16	
12	m			X						4	4	7	Cutaneous ureterostomy, UCN, cutaneous ureterostomy	3	4	15	7	
13	m			X						1	1	1	UCN	2	5	18	17	
14	f			X						3	3	5	Cutaneous ureterostomy	1	5	18	12	
15	m			X						1/12	1/12	1/12	Nephrostomy	1	†			Died 6 weeks post-op
16	f				X					3/12	3/12	5/12	Cutaneous ureterostomy	1	5	9	9	Awaiting renal transplantation
17	f					X				3	3	8	Ureteropyelostomy, renal transplantation	1	6	21	13	Cross renal dystopia
18	f						X			9	9	9	Nephrostomy	1	†			
19	f							X		2	2	9	Pyelolithotomy	2	2	22	20	Anal atresia, mother of one child
20	f								X	9	9	9	Anderson-Hynes pyeloplasty, dialysis	2	1	15	6	

[a] Score system: 1 = no urinary infections, free urinary drainage; 2 = recurrent urinary infections, free urinary drainage; 3 = recurrent urinary infections, impaired urinary drainage; 4 = compensated renal retention, creatinine >120 μmol/liter; 5 = dialysis; 6 = renal transplantation

Abbreviations: X = main diagnosis; Y = additional diagnosis; ARP = antireflux plasty; UCN = ureterocystoneostomy

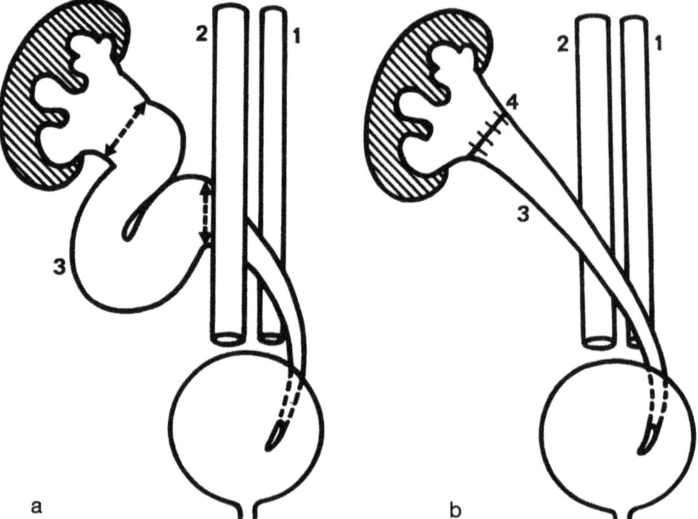

Fig. 1a, b. Cross-dystopia with retrocaval ureter: **a** anatomical situs; **b** state following antecaval displacement of the ureter, resection of ureteral kinking and pyeloureterostomy. *1,* Aorta; *2,* IVC; *3,* ureter before and after displacement; *4,* anastomosis

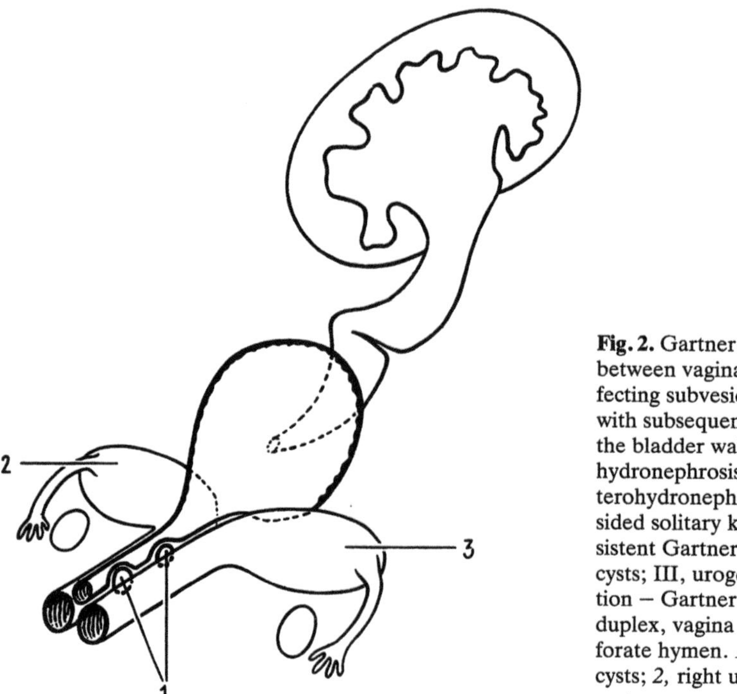

Fig. 2. Gartner duct cysts located between vagina and urethra, effecting subvesical obstruction with subsequent hypertrophy of the bladder wall and ureterohydronephrosis. Triad: I, Ureterohydronephrosis of the right-sided solitary kidney; II, persistent Gartner duct vaginal cysts; III, urogenital malformation − Gartner duct cysts, ureter duplex, vagina duplex, imperforate hymen. *1,* Gartner duct cysts; *2,* right ureter; *3,* left ureter

Table 2. Results of five operations for stenosis of the ureteropelvic junction in solitary kidneys

Operations performed	
Anderson-Hynes pyeloplasty	
Doing well 8 years post-op	1
Doing well 10 years post-op	1
Doing well 11 years post-op	1
Nephrostomy	
Spontaneous closure	1
Died	1

Table 3. Indications for nephrectomy resulting in secondary solitary kidney in 21 cases

Renal dysplasia	2
Hydronephrotic renal shrinkage	3
Cystic renal dysplasia (hypoplasia)	1
Suppurating pyelonephritis	1
Pyelonephritic renal shrinkage	7
Pyonephrosis with pelvic calculus	1
Pyonephrosis	4
Neurogenic bladder, pyelonephritis	1
Wilms' tumour	1

The finding of cross-dystopia in a solitary kidney with a retrocaval ureter (Krause and Piehl 1975; case 17 in Table 1) was made when the patient was already 8 years old. Immediately thereafter, the right ureter was displaced antecavally (Fig. 1). Five years following surgery, the child had to be dialysed for a period of 1 year because of renal decompensation. Renal transplantation was performed when the patient was 14. She did well for 7 years after this operation, but now, at 21 years of age, she has to be dialysed again.

The gartnerian cysts shown in Fig. 2 were not diagnosed during the lifetime of the patient. In 1964 we created a nephrostomy in the kidney, in which only a few millimetres of parenchyma were left. The girl died 3 years later of uraemia (Gdanietz 1964).

Cases 1–5 in Table 1 involved stenoses of the ureteropelvic junction. In three of them (cases 1, 2 and 4) an Anderson-Hynes pyeloplasty was performed, and in the remaining two, a nephrostomy (cases 3 and 5). Results are shown in Table 2.

Cases 9–15 in Table 1 involved ostial stenoses. Primary resection of the stenosis with subsequent reimplantation was possible in only one case; pathological changes of the upper urinary tract prevented this procedure in the others, in which recurrent urinary infections, extending to pyonephrosis, made free urinary drainage the first requirement. Using antimicrobials, it was essential to prevent further progression of renal insufficiency. Nevertheless, two of the patients (cases 13 and 14), now both 18 years old, require dialysis.

Two other patients (cases 11 and 12), now 15 and 25 years old, are in the state of compensated renal retention. One girl (case 9, aged 10 years) is in excellent condition 7 years following ureteral reimplantation, and one boy (case 10, aged 15 years) is doing well 14 years after ureteral reimplantation. An infant (case 15) died of pyonephrosis at the age of 6 weeks.

Secondary Solitary Kidneys ($n = 21$)

Due to loss of a kidney, 21 children had secondary solitary kidneys. Reasons for nephrectomy are shown in Table 3. Table 4 summarizes indications for surgery of

Table 4. Diagnoses, treatment and assessment in surgical interventions of secondary solitary kidneys

	Sex	Stenosis of ureteropelvic junction	Hydronephrosis	Double kidney	Vesicoureteral reflux	Ostial stenosis	Nephrolithiasis	Neurogenic bladder	Subvesical obstruction	Age at onset of disease (years)	Age at initiation of treatment (years)	Age at surgery (years)	Therapy	No. of operations	Assessment[a]	Age at follow-up (years)	Length of follow-up (years)	Remarks
1	m	X								3	3	4	Anderson-Hynes pyeloplasty	1	1	9	5	Contralateral Wilms' tumour, nephrectomy
2	f	X								1	3	3	Anderson-Hynes pyeloplasty	1	2	11	8	
3	f	X								8	8	9	Anderson-Hynes pyeloplasty	1	2	23	14	Mother of two children
4	f	X		Y	Y					2/12	7/12	7/12	Anderson-Hynes pyeloplasty	1	3	12	12	
5	m	X								4	4	4	Dialysis, nephrostomy, Fenger-plasty	2	4	22	18	
6	m		X		Y				Y	5/12	5/12	1	Nephrostomy, Y-V plasty, UCN, transplantation	3	6	13	13	
7	m			X	Y					4	4	8	Heminephrectomy	1	1	17	9	
8	f				X					2	2	7	Antireflux plasties	4	4	15	13	
9	m				Y	X				1	1	1	UCN	1	1	18	16	
10	f					X				3	3	3	Nephrostomy, cutaneous ureterostomy, Boari-plasty	3	1	22	19	

No.	Sex												Operation					Remarks
11	f						X			13	13	15	Ureterolithotomy	1	2	23	10	Mother of one child
12	f						X			3	3	10	Pyelolithotomy, ureterolithotomy	2	2	23	20	
13	m			Y			X	Y		4	14	16	Pyelolithotomy, ureterolithotomy, cutaneous ureterostomy	4	3	20	16	High post-traumatic paraplegia
14	m				Y		X	Y	Y	1	1	15	Cutaneous ureterostomy	1	4	18	17	Myelomeningocele, cerebral damage
15	f				Y			X		2	2	4	UCN	1	†			Died 2 years post-op
16	m								X	1/12	1/12	2/12	Cutaneous ureterostomy	1	3	1	1	
17	m								X	5/12	5/12	5/12	Nephrostomy, UCN, cutaneous ureterostomy	3	3	5	5	
18	m				Y				X	2/12	2/12	3/12	Cutaneous ureterostomy, UCN, cutaneous ureterostomy	4	3	13	13	Cerebral damage in infancy
19	m	Y			Y				X	2/12	2/12	2/12	Nephrostomy, TUR, UCN, Fenger-plasty	11	4	15	15	Operated elsewhere
20	m								X	1/12	1/12	4/12	Cutaneous ureterostomy	1	4	6	6	Nephrolithiasis
21	m				Y				X	1	1	1	ARP, cutaneous ureterostomy	2	5	19	18	

[a] Score: (see Table 1)

Abbreviations: X = main diagnosis; Y = additional diagnosis; UCN = ureterocystoneostomy; TUR = transurethral resection; ARP = antireflux plasty

Table 5. Results of surgical interventions in primary and secondary kidneys

Score[a]	Primary solitary kidney			Secondary solitary kidney		
	No. of patients	% (total $n = 20$)		No. of patients	(total $n = 21$)	
1	3	15		4	19.05	
2	6	30	good results in 55%	4	19.05	good results in 61.9%
3	2	10		5	23.81	
4	2	10		5	23.81	
5	3	15		1	4.76	
6	1	5	poor results in 45%	1	4.76	poor results in 38.1%
Died	3	15		1	4.76	

[a] Score: (see Table 1)

the remaining kidney, as well as further treatment and assessment. One child (case 19) with subvesical obstruction endured 11 operations before transferral to our clinic.

Discussion

The fate of children with solitary kidneys depends crucially on the underlying disease. In secondary solitary kidneys we found that several different urological diseases were present simultaneously, already having damaged both organs. Thus, the necessary operation in the remaining kidney was carried out in a predamaged organ. These drawbacks impaired the prognosis. If we consider the courses in the different diagnostic groups, our study revealed that subvesical obstructions have the poorest prognosis due to secondary pathological changes. Five of six children now carry a permanent cutaneous ureterostomy as a result of severe associated malformations, in some cases following one to four corrective operations. Stenoses of the ureteropelvic junction have a better prognosis. Four of five children developed well (cases 1–4 in Table 4), one is in a state of compensated renal retention (case 5 in Table 4). These patients now range in age from 9 to 23 years; one woman (case 3 in Table 4) has two healthy children.

References

Gdanietz K (1964) Beitrag zur Hydronephrose im Kindesalter infolge Harnobstruktion durch Gartnersche Gangzysten bei kombinierter Urogenitalmißbildung. Zentralbl Chir 89:1302–1310

Krause I, Piehl G (1975) Retrokavalureter und gekreuzte Dystopie bei Einnierigkeit. Zentralbl Chir 100:503–506

Bladder Shrinkage as a Complication
of Long-Term Supravesical Urinary Diversion
in Children with Solitary Kidneys

M. Gharib and R. Engelskirchen

Summary

Failures in the treatment of terminal ureteral stenosis are not seldom burdened by considerable bladder shrinkage, particularly in infants. Congenital anomalies of the urinary tract such as bilaterally ectopic ureteral ostia can also lead to bladder shrinkage, even in newborns.

Using examples from our patient series, we discuss problems of contracted bladder in children and describe a method of continuous bladder distention by means of catheters with different balloon volumes and a simultaneous, intermittent, hydrostatic bladder dilatation. This method enables reintegration of a bladder which has been excluded from the urinary drainage system for a long period of time into the urinary tract, even in complicated cases, thus avoiding a permanent supravesical urinary diversion.

Zusammenfassung

Fehlschläge in der Behandlung der terminalen Harnleiterstenose sind gerade im Säuglingsalter nicht selten mit einer erheblichen Blasenschrumpfung belastet. Auch angeborene Anomalien der ableitenden Harnwege wie beidseits ektop mündende Ureteren können schon bei Neugeborenen zu einer Schrumpfblase führen.

Anhand von Beispielen aus unserem Krankengut wird die Problematik der kontrakten Harnblase bei Kindern dargelegt und die Methode der kontinuierlichen Blasendistension mit Kathetern unterschiedlicher Ballonvolumina sowie gleichzeitiger intermittierender hydrostatischer Dehnung der Harnblase vorgestellt. Mit diesem Verfahren ist es auch in kompliziert gelagerten Fällen oft noch möglich, eine langzeit ausgeschaltete Harnblase in das ableitende Harnwegssystem zu reintegrieren und damit eine definitive supravesicale Harnableitung zu umgehen.

Résumé

Les échecs lors du traitement de la sténose terminale des voies urinaires se compliquent fréquemment d'un rétrécissement considérable de la vessie, surtout dans

Paediatric Surgical Clinic, Children's Hospital of Cologne, Department of Paediatric Urology, Amsterdamerstr. 59, D-5000 Köln 60, Federal Republic of Germany

Progress in Pediatric Surgery, Vol. 23
Ed. by L. Spitz et al.
© Springer-Verlag Berlin Heidelberg 1989

le cas de nourrissons. Les anomalies congénitales des voies urinaires excrétrices telles qu'uretères implantés de façon ectopique et bilatérale peuvent provoquer chez les nouveaux-nés un r étrécissement de la vessie.

Nous relatons des exemples illustrant les problèmes associés à la contraction de la vessie chez les enfants et décrivons une méthode de distension continuelle de la vessie à l'aide de cathéters à ballonnets accompagneé d'une dilatation intermittente hydrostatique de la vessie. Cette procédure permet souvent, même dans les cas compliqués, le raccord de la vessie aux voies excrétrices et d'éviter ainsi une dérivation définitive supravésicale de l'urine.

Bladder shrinkage in children can be due, on the one hand, to congenital, bilateral, terminal ureteral stenoses or to bilaterally ectopic ureteral ostia and, on the other hand, to a long-term supravesical urinary diversion. Supravesical urinary diversion becomes necessary mostly following ureteral reimplantation for treatment of recurrent stenosis, particularly in children with solitary kidneys. Other causes of bladder shrinkage, such as tuberculosis or irradiation fibrosis, are of minor importance in paediatric urology. Tanagho (1974) correctly emphasizes the particular therapeutic problems arising from congenital bladder shrinkage.

Since the first description by Bumpus in 1930 (cited by Tankó and Kálmán 1984), hydrostatic bladder distention has been a well-known procedure for improving bladder capacity; it has been applied chiefly in the treatment of unstable bladder (Delaere et al. 1980) and interstitial cystitis (Beer et al. 1986) and for certain tumours (Helmstein 1972) in recent years. In order to remind the reader of this very adequate method for preserving or restoring the function of a contracted bladder in children we feel it justified to report on our experience with combined hydrostatic bladder dilatation in children.

Method

In infants with primary bladder hypoplasia, catheters of increasing volume are inserted transurethrally into the bladder, beginning with CH 6 (balloon volume 5–6 ml) and continuing to CH 10 (volume 15–20 ml). The balloon is continuously inflated with saline solution; the fractional instillation of body-warm saline solution allows for inflation of the balloon to more than its stated maximal capacity. Additionally, the bladder is filled three to five times a day with warm saline solution under a hydrostatic pressure of 40–60 cm H_2O to achieve an extension of the bladder which goes beyond the basic extension achieved by the inflated balloon. At the same time, the bladder mucosa kept continuously moist, thus improving the elasticity of the muscle and the connective fibers.

In children with gross dilatation of the proximal urethra due to posterior urethral valves the catheters are inserted suprapubically, since otherwise the blocked balloon would be displaced from the rigid bladder into the dilated urethra and a dilatation effect on the bladder would be impossible. Another advantage to

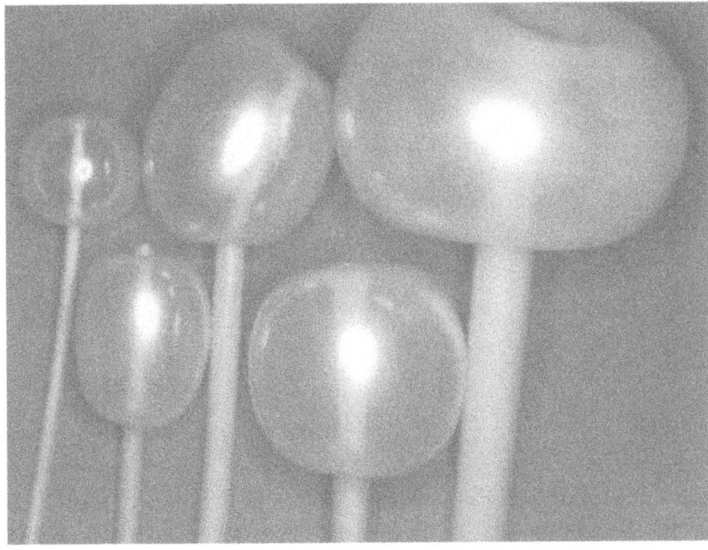

Fig. 1. Bladder catheters of various sizes with balloon volumes ranging from 7 to 80 ml

this is that larger catheters (CH 18, balloon volume 50–80 ml) can later be inserted into the bladder in older infants (Fig. 1).

The duration of distention treatment prior to ureteral reimplantation is from 2 months in newborns to 6 months in older children with long-term bladder diversion, depending on the basic situation and the age. When a bladder capacity of 40 ml in newborns, 80 ml in older infants and 150 ml in older children is reached, a unilateral ureteral reimplantation can be carried out, effecting a permanent volume capacity and moistening of the bladder wall, which in turn further increases bladder capacity.

Case Reports

1. The first boy presented 1 day after birth with urosepsis due to highly impaired urinary drainage, which was caused by posterior urethral valves. He had severe bilateral hydronephrosis with reflux stenoses of both terminal ureters. Secondary to repeated bilateral nephrostomies a loop fistula was created on the left side, and the right kidney was removed at the age of 6 months, following entire loss of function. The child was transferred to us after having had supravesical urinary diversion for 10 months. At that time he had a contracted bladder with a maximal filling capacity of less than 10 ml and a reflux into the right ureteral stump which remained after nephrectomy. The balloon catheter with a volume of 3 ml could be placed only in the proximal urethra (Fig. 2). In the meantime, the left reflux stenosis had scarred to a complete ostial stenosis, as was shown by antegrade contrast radiography via the loop fistula (Fig. 3). Bladder dilatation, performed via suprapubically inserted catheters, had to be carried out for reintegration of the bladder into the urinary drainage system. After distention treatment using catheters with increasing volumes and additional bladder lavage for 3 months a bladder capacity of 50 ml was achieved. At this time we completely resected the posterior urethral valves and reimplanted

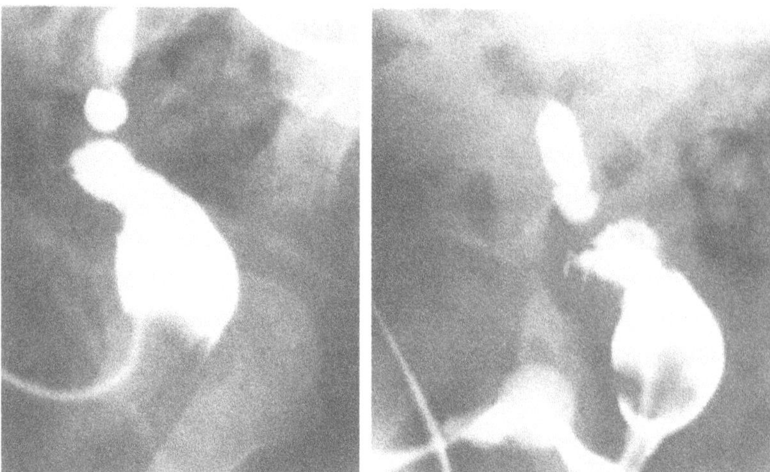

Fig. 2. Contracted bladder in an infant secondary to 10 months of supravesical urinary diversion for bilateral reflux stenoses in posterior urethral valves. The balloon of the catheter with a volume of 3 ml is placed in the proximal urethra; the detrusor is maximally contracted. Refluxing ureteral stump left after nephrectomy is seen on the right

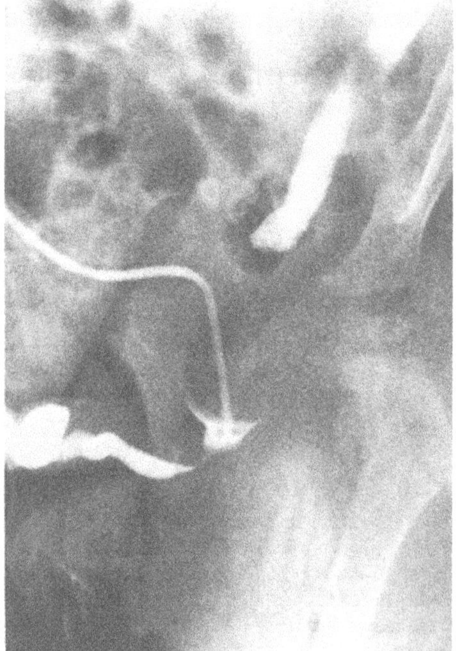

Fig. 3. Case 1: antegrade contrast radiograph of the completely obstructed terminal ureter via nephrostomy. Distention catheter with a balloon volume of 3 ml is inserted suprapubically

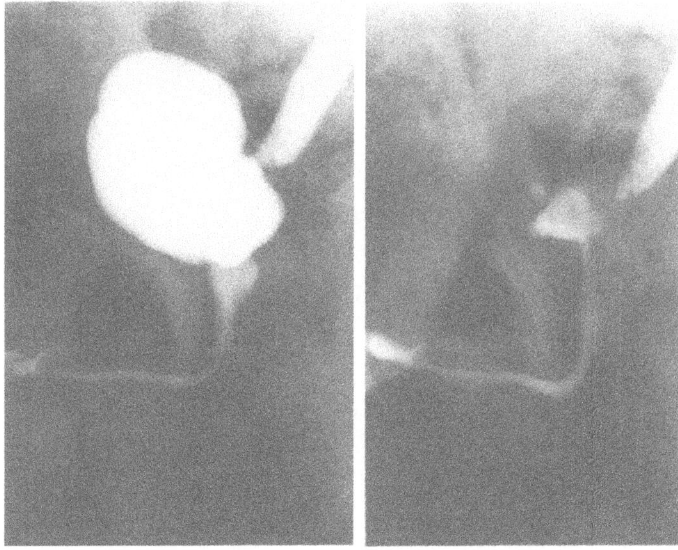

Fig. 4. Case 1: MCU 6 months after reimplantation of the left ureter and excision of the right ureteral stump. Normal bladder capacity; nearly complete voiding; still VUR on the left side

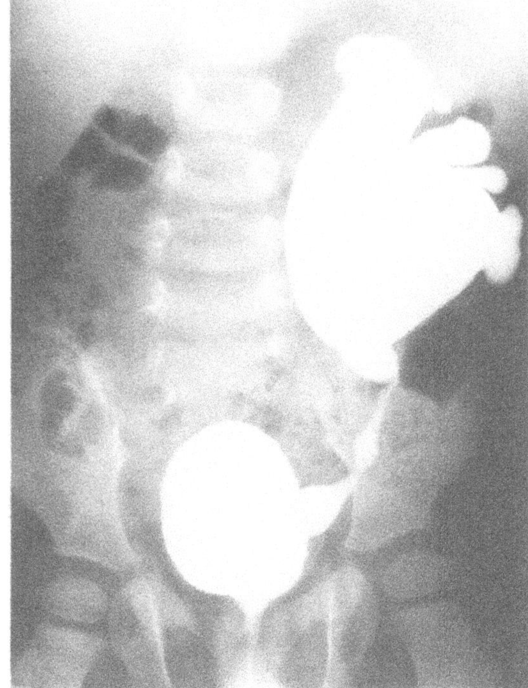

Fig. 5. Case 2: MCU in a 9-month-old boy with posterior urethral valves, massive left-sided VUR and ostial stenosis on the right side

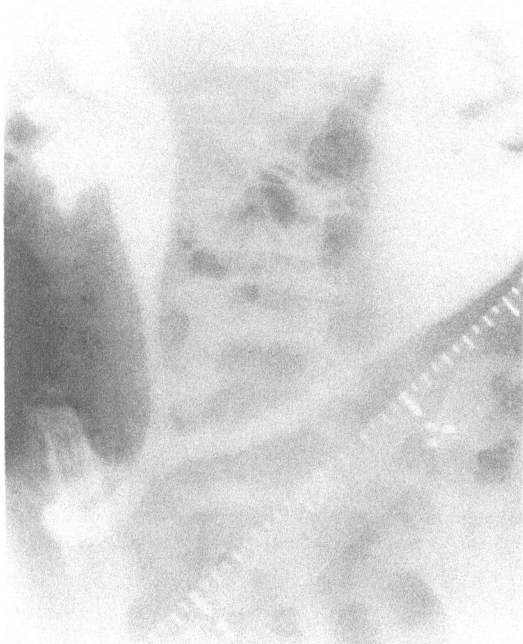

Fig. 6. Case 2: retrograde contrast radiograph of the urinary collecting system 6 years after Y-uretero-ureterocutaneostomy

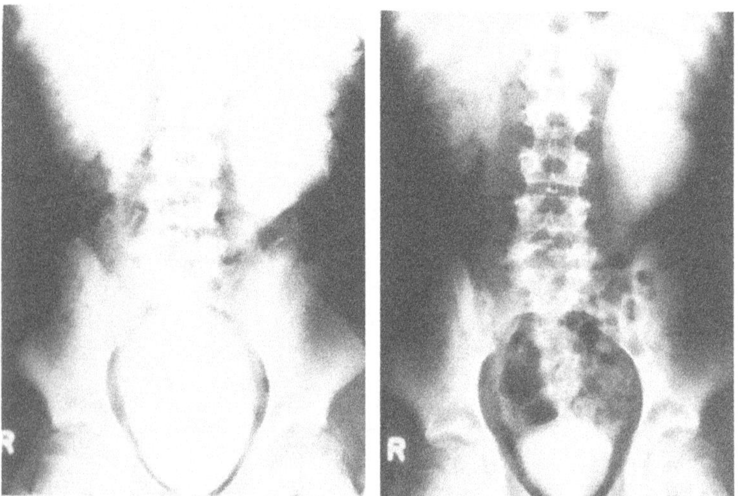

Fig. 7. Case 2: i.v. pyelogram following 6 months of bladder distention and reimplantation before *(left)* and after *(right)* micturition. Bladder shows normal size and good contractility

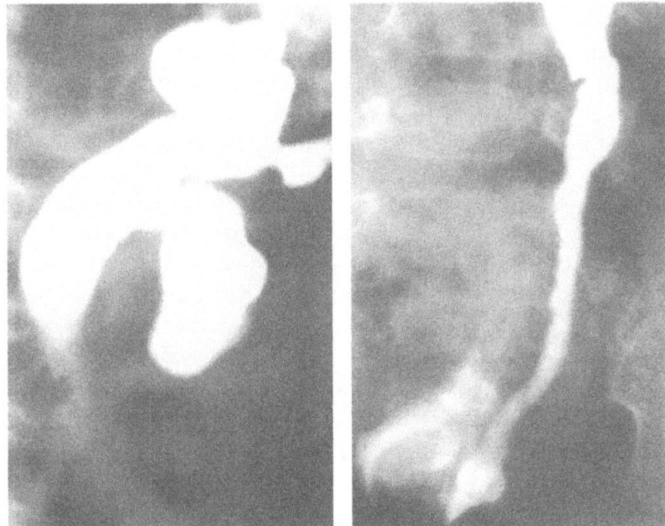

Fig. 8. Case 3: contracted bladder secondary to double failure of reimplantation of a single ureter on the left side in a 2-year-old boy. Cicatricial stricture of the terminal ureter; bladder capacity 20 ml

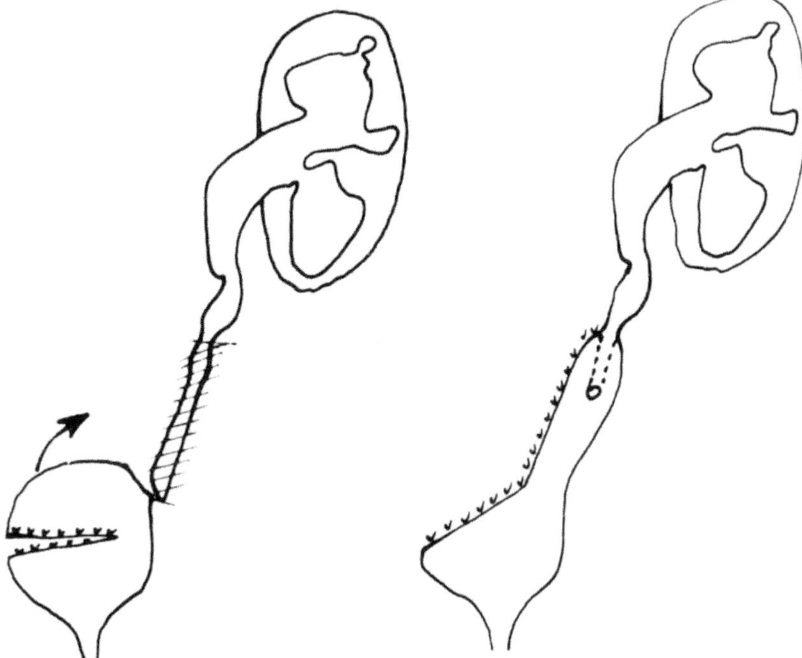

Fig. 9. Case 3: corrective bladder surgery for replacement of the distal ureter

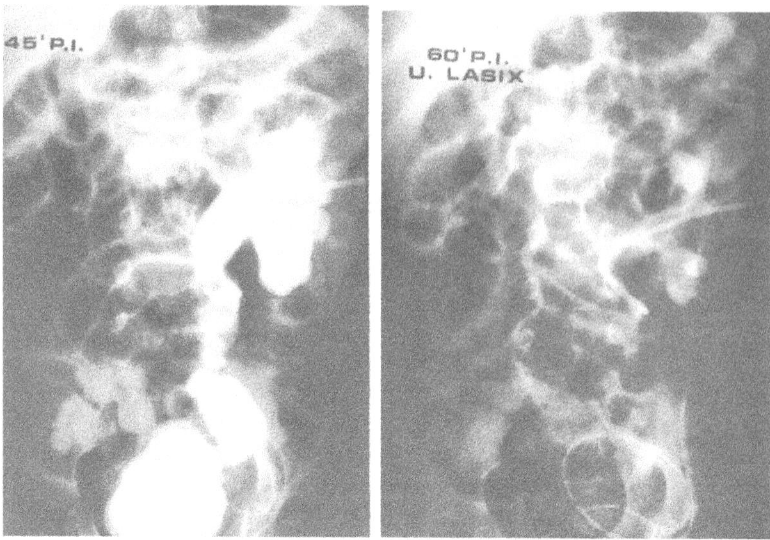

Fig. 10. Case 3: i.v. pyelogram 3 weeks after reimplantation, with prompt drainage of the contrast medium after administration of furosemide

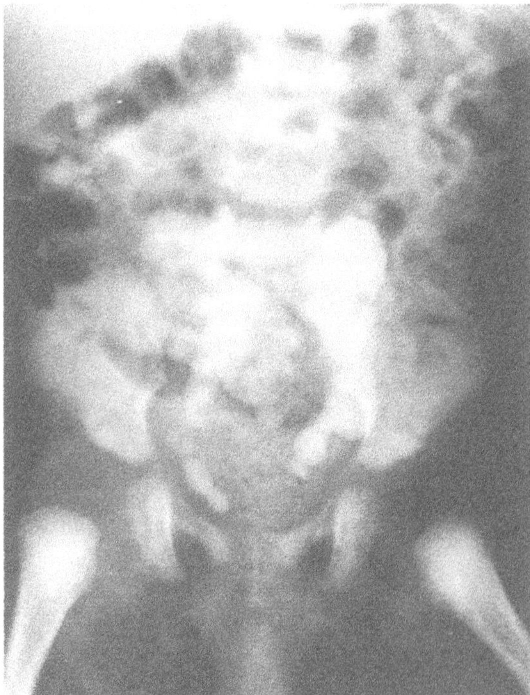

Fig. 11. Case 4: i.v. pyelogram in a 4-week-old girl with both ureters ending ectopically in the vagina. Note lack of bladder exposure

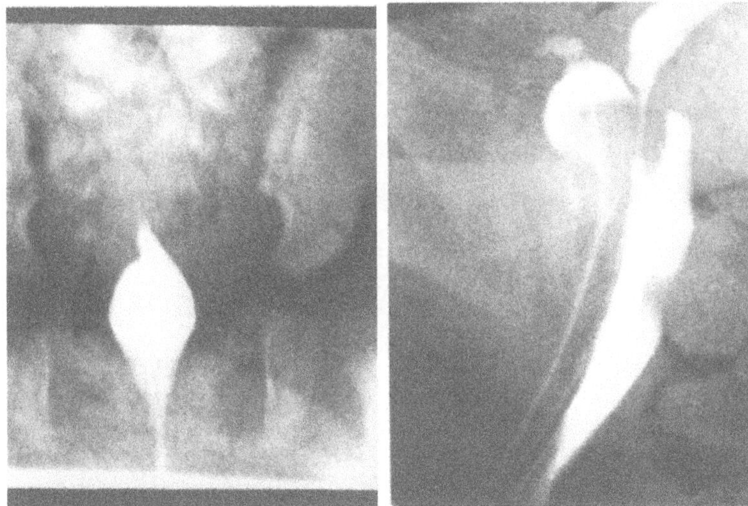

Fig. 12. Case 4: retrograde filling of the bladder (balloon volume, 3 ml), one of the ectopically ending ureters, and the vagina

the left ureter. Micturition cystourethrography (MCU) performed 6 months later revealed a nearly normal bladder size with vesicoureteral reflux as well as complete voiding (Fig. 4).

With permanent antibiotic prophylaxis the boy has been free of urinary infections since then and has unimpaired micturition. An antireflux plasty has not been necessary so far, since no further urinary infections have occurred, scintigraphic renal function tests have shown consistent performance of the damaged organ for 2 years, and half-yearly MCU checks reveal decreasing VUR. In case of new urinary infections, an antireflux plasty according to Gregoir is planned.

2. With the second boy, and MCU at the age of 9 months revealed a massive VUR on the left side with posterior urethral valves and a right-sided terminal ureteral stenosis (Fig. 5). Following repeated failure with reimplantations on both sides, the last on the left by a Boari-plasty, a definitive Y-uretero-ureterocutaneostomy was carried out when the boy was 3 years old. Nine years later, retrograde contrast radiography revealed gross dilatation of both renal cavities and considerably shortened ureters (Fig. 6). At this time the bladder, which had been diverted for a long period, had a maximum capacity of 20 ml. This could be increased to 150 ml by intermittent bladder dilatation with transurethral balloon catheters and regular saline lavage up to a maximal hydrostatic pressure of 100 cm H_2O. This enabled us to reimplant the right distal ureter without prosthesis into the bladder that had been inactivated for 9 years (Fig. 7). Later MCU checks showed a bladder of age-corresponding size without VUR and unimpaired micturition.

3. Our third patient, a boy, also had posterior urethral valves with secondary bilateral hydronephrosis. He presented with urosepis and was aided by supravesical urinary diversion. When he was 4 weeks old, a transurethral valve resection, ureteral reimplantation on the left side and excision of the scintigraphically functionless right kidney were performed in one session. Because of recurrent ureteral stenosis on the left side, a cutaneous nephrostomy had to be established. After the second reimplantation of the left ureter 8 months later, another stenosis developed; thus, the bladder was inactivated for 2 years. When the boy was transferred to us at this age, he had a stenosis of the left distal ureter covering a long distance and no peristalsis. The bladder had a maximal capacity of 20 ml (Fig. 8). Capacity could be increased to 80 ml by means of dilatation treatment, enabling us to perform a renewed ureteral reimplantation. The long stenosis had to be resected in order to avoid further recurrence. To bridge the long ureteral gap, we divided the bladder laterally and brought the upper part of the bladder to the ureter, following a Psoas-Hitch

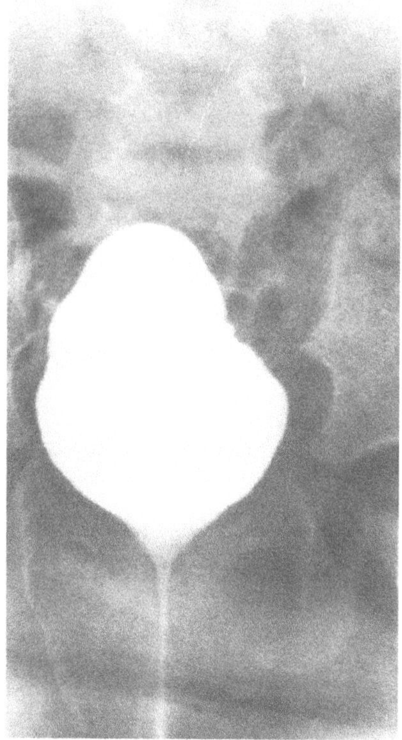

Fig. 13. Case 4: MCU 3 months after unilateral reimplantation, which was performed following 5 months of bladder distention. Age-correspondent bladder capacity, no VUR

procedure (Fig. 9). An i.v. pyelogram performed 3 weeks postoperatively revealed prompt drainage of the upper urinary tract after administration of furosemide, and we could finally remove the nephrostomy catheter after more than 2 years (Fig. 10).

4. Considerable dilatation of both renal cavities and ureters was noted sonographically in a newborn girl who was transferred to us because of anal atresia. Delimitation of the urinary bladder was missing on the ultrasound picture. An i.v. pyelogram performed when the girl was 4 weeks old confirmed bilateral hydronephrosis and the missing bladder exposure (Fig. 11). Retrograde contrast radiography revealed a highly hypoplastic bladder with a maximal capacity of 3 ml, due to the fact that both ureters ended ectopically in the vestibulum vaginae; one of them is shown here (Fig. 12). Careful bladder dilatation and unilateral ureteral reimplantation were performed when the girl was 5 months old, and a control MCU performed 3 months postoperatively showed normal, age-corresponding bladder size, enabling us to reimplant the other ureter without difficulties. Since then the girl has been free of urinary infections, and she has no VUR (Fig. 13).

Discussion

Shrinkage of the bladder in children is most frequently due to long-term detrusor inactivation, which results either from ectopically ending ureters or from long-term suprapubic urinary diversion. Nephrostomies or cutaneous ureterostomies are established mostly because better therapeutic concepts are lacking for bilateral terminal ureteral stenoses or infravesical blockage of urinary drainage in newborns. If shrinkage due to inactivity of the bladder results, it is generally not because of loss of detrusor muscle, but rather because of an increase of connective tissue between the contracted smooth muscle bundles. Normally, the texture of detrusor muscle is maintained, as could be shown in biopsy specimens taken from contracted infant bladders. The situation is different when recurrent inflammatory episodes attack the bladder: according to Lome et al. (1972), transmural fibrosis develops, rendering all attempts at dilatation impossible. For seven of his 30 children with contracted bladders a permanent suprapubic urinary diversion therefore had to be established. He reports a permanent normalization of bladder capacity if ureteral reimplantation can be carried out successfully; this is in accordance with our own experience.

In contrast to Tankó and Kálmán, who perform bladder distention with adults under epidural anaesthesia and with children under general anaesthesia, we prefer the more time-consuming, but more careful procedure of continuous bladder dilatation without anaesthesia; this has also been applied successfully by Perlmutter et al. (1975).

To prevent bladder shrinkage and its complications, long-term diversion of the bladder must be avoided, even in severe cases. This means that surgical correction must be carried out as early as in infancy, as is rightly emphasized by Hendren (1970). However, an adequate technique is essential to avoid any risk of recurrent stenosis following ureteral reimplantation. For this reason, a modified Cohen procedure, which we have performed successfully for years, is particularly suited in newborns and infants (Gharib et al., in press).

If one is nevertheless confronted with a child who has a contracted bladder, a permanent supravesical urinary diversion is not indicated, in our experience, unless an adequate hydrostatic bladder dilatation has been tried. Careful, long-lasting, intermittent bladder dilatation makes it possible to reintegrate the bladder into the urinary drainage system and thus avoid a permanent suprapubic urinary diversion.

References

Beer M, Marx FJ, Schmiedt E (1986) Konservative Therapie der chronischen interstitiellen Zystitis durch hydrostatische Ballondilatation and adjuvante Pentosan-Polysulfat-Medikation. Akt Urol 17:119–123

Delaere KPJ, Debruyne FMJ, Michiels HGE, Moonen WA (1980) Prolonged bladder distension in the management of the unstable bladder. J Urol 124:334–337

Gharib M, Engelskirchen R, Ebel K-D (1989) Correction of terminal ureteral obstruction in the neonate and infant: surgical technique and functional results. Ped Surg Int (in press)

Helmstein K (1972) Treatment of bladder carcinoma by a hydrostatic pressure technique: report of 43 cases. Br J Urol 44:434–450

Hendren WH (1970) A new approach to infants with severe obstructive uropathy: early complete reconstruction. J Pediatr Surg 5:184–199

Lome LG, Howat JM, Williams DI (1972) The temporarily defunctionalized bladder in children. J Urol 107:469–472

Perlmutter AD, Gonzales ET Jr, Christensen LC (1975) The contracted bladder and ureteral diversion – one approach to reconstruction: a case report. J Urol 113:716–718

Tanagho EA (1974) Congenitally obstructed bladders: fate after prolonged defunctionalization. J Urol 111:102–109

Tankó A, Kálmán J (1984) Distensionsbehandlung der Harnblase. Urologe [Ausg A] 23:226–228

Problems in Severe Bilateral Urinary Tract Anomalies

O. H. Nielsen and J. Thorup

Summary

Management of children with severe infravesical or bilateral ureterovesical obstruction with or without reflux is difficult. Our experience over 10 years includes 29 such children, 19 of whom presented in the first 3 months of life. At the time of diagnosis, 13 had severe disturbance of renal function.

There were two deaths. Five children have severe and two a moderate reduction of renal function; twenty good renal function.

There were ten nephrectomies and four heminephrectomies. Seven patients had a temporary and eight a permanent urinary diversion. However, four of the latter were later undiverted.

Removal of an obstruction is not always followed by full restitution of function. It seems probable that renal dysplasia and developmental injury to the uterovesical musculature set a limit to the therapeutic possibilities.

Careful management is important, especially in neonatal cases, where extensive reconstructive procedures are technically demanding and the rate of complications is high.

Zusammenfassung

Die Behandlungsprobleme bei infravesikaler oder doppelseitiger ureterovesikaler Obstruktion mit oder ohne Reflux sind groß. Unsere Erfahrungen über zehn Jahre umfassen 29 Kinder, von denen 19 unter drei Monaten alt waren. Zur Zeit der Diagnose hatten 13 schwere Nierenfunktionsstörungen.

Davon sind 2 gestorben. Fünf haben schwere und 2 leichte Reduktion der Nierenfunktion. Gute Nierenfunktion haben 20.

Zehn Nephrektomien und 4 Heminephrektomien sind ausgeführt worden. Sieben Patienten haben temporäre und 8 permanente Harnableitung bekommen. Doch sind davon 4 später wieder rückoperiert worden.

Der Behebung einer Obstruktion folgt nicht immer eine völlige funktionelle Restitution. Wahrscheinlich ist, daß sowohl renale Dysplasie als auch Schädigung der ureterovesikalen Muskulatur häufig die Möglichkeiten der Therapie begrenzen.

University Clinic of Paediatric Surgery, Rigshospitalet, DK-2100 Copenhagen Ø, Denmark

Progress in Pediatric Surgery, Vol. 23
Ed. by L. Spitz et al.
© Springer-Verlag Berlin Heidelberg 1989

Eine wohlgeplante Behandlungsstrategie ist wichtig, vor allem bei Säuglingen, bei denen große rekonstruktive Eingriffe mit technischen Schwierigkeiten und häufig mit Komplikationen verbunden sind.

Résumé

Le traitement des obstructions infravésicales ou urétérovésicales bilatérales avec ou sans reflux pose des problèmes considérables. En l'espace de 10 ans, nous avons traité 29 enfants dont 19 âgés de moins de trois mois. Dans 13 cas, le diagnostique avait révélé une altération grave de la fonction rénale.

Il y a eu deux décès. La fonction rénale est gravement altérée dans cinq cas, légèrement insuffisante dans deux cas et bonne dans 20 cas.

Dix néphrectomies et quatre héminéphrectomies ont été pratiquées. Pour sept patients, il y a eu une dérivation temporaire de l'urine et une dérivation permanente chez huit patients avec toutefois une réintégration dans quatre cas. La levée de l'obstruction ne suffit pas toujours à rétablir complètement la fonction rénale. Il est probable que la dysplasie rénale et les atteintes d'origine embryonnaire de la musculature urétérovésicale limitent les possibilités thérapeutiques.

L'ensemble de la thérapie y compris les gestes thérapeutiques doivent être soigneusement pesés, surtout quand il s'agit de nouveaux-nés, car les technqiues de reconstruction étendue sont extrêmement délicates et le taux de complications élevé.

Optimal management of children with severe bilateral or infravesical urinary tract obstruction is important. The condition is a serious threat to renal function, and such patients make a substantial contribution to the group of candidates for dialysis and renal transplantation (Barratt and Baillod 1982).

Material and Methods

During the 10-year period 1976–1985, 29 children (23 boys and six girls) with severe bilateral urinary tract anomalies were treated at the Department of Paediatric Surgery, Rigshospitalet. Their age at the time of diagnosis was 0–3 years (median: 6 weeks). Nineteen children presented within the first 3 months of life. In Table 1 the patients have been listed in six diagnostic groups. The group "Others" includes two children with bilateral duplication and combinations of ectopic ureter, ureterocele, reflux and ureteral obstruction, one girl with myelomeningocele and severe neurogenic bladder dysfunction, one girl with adrenogenital syndrome, urogenital sinus with hydrometrocolpos, unilateral single ectopic ureterocele and contralateral reflux, and one boy with oesophageal atresia and a urethroanal H-fistula.

The patients were evaluated with ultrasonic scan, intravenous pyelography, micturition cystourethrography and renal scintiscan. The renal function was evaluated on the basis of renography, DTPA clearance and creatinine clearance.

Table 1. Diagnoses in 29 cases of bilateral urinary tract anomalies

Megaloureter with bilateral vesicoureteral reflux	9
Megaloureter with bilateral vesicoureteral obstruction	4
Megaloureter with unilateral reflux and contralateral obstruction	3
Urethral valves	6
Prune-belly syndrome	2
Others	5

Table 2. Operative procedures in 29 cases of bilateral urinary tract anomalies

Ureteroneocystostomy	31
Nephrectomy	10
Heminephrectomy	4
Urethral valve resection	6
Temporary diversion	7
Permanent diversion	8
Undiversion	4

The operative procedures employed are listed in Table 2. In principle, they were directed against the primary pathology. Temporary diversion was not used as a routine, but only when indicated by the combination of severe obstruction and infection. The indication for nephrectomy was loss of function to a value below 10% of total renal function.

Only major operations are listed, and the number of procedures, not ureters, are counted. The majority of ureteral reimplantations were bilateral. Resection of valves was done transurethrally, in three neonatal cases via a perineal urethrostomy.

Results

In the group of refluxing megaloureters all patients had ureteroneocystostomies, in one case with ureteral tapering. In five cases a reoperation was needed; two of these children had neuromuscular bladder dysfunction. There were no nephrectomies in this group, but two patients with initially poor renal function are on the verge of renal insufficiency. One of them had a permanent diversion but is now undiverted on a self-catheterization regime.

Three of the four patients with obstructed megaloureters presented with severely reduced renal function. All had ureteroneocystostomies but were later diverted. Two kidneys have been removed. One patient has been undiverted and another is being prepared for undiversion. Two have severely reduced and one moderately reduced renal function.

One of the patients with megaloureters with mixed obstruction and reflux presented with poor renal function which is since somewhat improved. All three of these patients had ureteroneocystostomies. Two kidneys were later removed — both on the refluxing side. The third boy now has a Boari flap on the refluxing side.

Three of the six boys with urethral valves had had a prenatal diagnosis of urinary tract dilatation. Two others presented in the neonatal period and the last at the age of 6 months. His valves, however, were found and resected much later. One boy died at the age of 2 months of severe bilateral renal dysplasia. Two boys had bilateral and one unilateral reflux; all three underwent nephrectomy. The outflow has been normalized in the five survivors, although in two cases urethral stricture required several internal urethrotomies, and ultimately urethroplasty in one. The remaining kidney function is good in all.

One of the boys with prune-belly syndrome also had severely dysplastic kidneys. He died at the age of 3 months. The other boy, in whom urinary tract dilatation was discovered prenatally, has had one dysplastic kidney removed. The function of the other kidney is reduced. Its ureter has been reimplanted twice, and it is vented through a Soper-ureterostomy.

In the group of "Others", one boy with bilateral duplication had two heminephroureterectomies, and a girl had one hemi- and one total nephroureterectomy. The girl with myelomeningocele had massive bilateral reflux and received a urinary diversion because of recurrent infections and incipient loss of renal function on one side. She has now been undiverted and is on a self-catheterization regime. The girl with adrenogenital syndrome had a neonatal laparotomy elsewhere, caused by her hydrometrocolpos. She later underwent a left nephrectomy with excision of the single ectopic ureterocele, right ureteroneocystostomy and vaginoplasty. The boy with a urethroanal fistula underwent urethral reconstruction, but since the function of his large bladder and wide ureters was poor he later received a diversion. Although the two patients with ureteral duplication presented with infection and reduced renal function, they both now have satisfactory renal function.

The summarized results for the entire group of 29 patients are: two deaths, 13 nephrectomies, four heminephrectomies, four remaining diversions, five patients with severe and two with moderate reduction of renal function — i.e. 27 survivors, 22 of whom have a good quality of life.

Discussion

Children with severe bilateral urinary tract anomalies are a highly selected group, dominated by boys. Their lesions are almost exclusively located at or below bladder level. Nonetheless, it is a highly heterogeneous group, from a pathological point of view. Normal urinary transport is often difficult to attain, and it seems probable that the muscular tissue of the ureters and bladder may be poorly developed or damaged in many cases, as a consequence of dilatation (Hanna et al.

1977). Developmental injury may also be the cause of the poor renal function, leading to many nephrectomies, or in the most severe cases to early death (Diamond et al. 1984). In the survivors, a clinical distinction between renal dysplasia and pyelonephritic atrophy is mostly impossible.

Early diagnosis and optimal management therefore remain extremely important in order to prevent additional functional damage. The majority of these patients present during the first months of life, and an increasing number are being identified prenatally (Kramer 1983). Extensive urinary tract reconstruction in neonates is technically demanding, and the rate of complications is high. This group of patients will remain one of the greatest challenges to paediatric urologists.

References

Barratt TM, Baillod RA (1982) Chronic renal failure and regular dialysis. In: Williams DI, Johnston JH (eds) Paediatric urology, 2nd edn. Butterworth, London, pp 37–47
Diamond DA, Sanders R, Jeffs RD (1984) Fetal hydronephrosis: considerations regarding urological intervention. J Urol 131:1155–1159
Hanna MK, Jeffs RD, Sturgess JM, Barkin M (1977) Ureteral structure and ultrastructure: the dilated ureter, clinico-pathological correlation. J Urol 117:28–32
Kramer SA (1983) Current status of fetal intervention for congenital hydronephrosis. J Urol 130:641–646

Double Ureter in Children: Surgical Management

M. H. Kheradpir and E. Bodaghi

Summary

Among 25 cases of double ureter which required surgical treatment, six were accompanied by ureterocele. Interpelvic anastomosis was performed in two cases with uretero-ureteral reflux. En bloc reimplantation was performed for ten double ureters, three of which had common ureteral orifice with reflux in both ureters. In three other cases there was a common segment with low bifurcation and uretero-ureteral reflux which had to be excised in order to create two ureteral orifices in the bladder.

Heminephrectomy with excision of the ureterocele combined with a simultaneous reimplantation of the ipsilateral ureter was performed in three cases. These cases were accompanied by a large ureterocele and reflux in the ipsilateral ureter. Upper-pole nephrectomy and partial ureterectomy without excision of the stump and ureterocele was performed in one case of small ureterocele without reflux. Excision of the ureterocele combined with en bloc reimplantation was performed in one case with relatively well preserved renal tissues. Follow-up results were satisfactory in the majority of the cases.

Zusammenfassung

Sechs der 25 Fälle von Ureter Duplex, die chirurgisch behandelt wurden, zeigten auch eine Ureterozele. In zwei Fällen mit uretero-uretralem Reflux wurde im Beckenraum eine Anastomose durchgeführt. In 10 Fällen von Ureter Duplex wurde eine Reimplantation "en bloc" durchgeführt. Drei davon hatten eine gemeinsame Ureteröffnung mit Reflux in beide Ureteren. Bei drei anderen Fällen fand sich ein gemeinsames Segment mit tiefangelegter Gabelung und uretero-urethralem Reflux. Sie mußte exzidiert werden, um zwei ureterale Öffnungen in der Blase anzulegen.

In drei Fällen wurde eine Heminephrektomie mit Exzision der Ureterozele und gleichzeitiger Reimplantation des gleichseitigen Ureters vorgenommen. In drei anderen Fällen zeigte sich eine ausgedehnte Ureterozele mit Reflux in den gleichseitigen Ureter. In einem Fall mit begrenzter Ureterozele ohne Reflux

University Clinic Children's Hospital of Teheran, Department of Paediatric Surgery and Paediatric Nephrology, Teheran, Iran

Progress in Pediatric Surgery, Vol. 23
Ed. by L. Spitz et al.
© Springer-Verlag Berlin Heidelberg 1989

wurde eine Teilnephrektomie im oberen Bereich und eine Teilureterektomie ohne Entfernen des Stumpfes und der Ureterozele vorgenommen. In einem Fall mit relativ gut erhaltenem Nierengewebe wurden eine Exzision der Ureterozele und Reimplantation "en bloc" durchgeführt. Die weitere Beobachtung zeigte in den meisten Fällen zufriedenstellende Ergebnisse.

Résumé

Six des 25 cas d'uretère double ayant subi un traitement chirugical présantaient aussi une urétérocèle. Dans deux cas avec reflux urétéro-urétéral, on pratiqua une anastomose intrapelvienne. Une réimplantation en bloc fut faite dans dix cas d'urétére double, dont trois avaient un orifice urétéral commun avec reflux dans les deux urétéres. Dans trois autres cas, il y avait un segment commun avec bifurcation basse et reflux urétéro-urétéral, qui fit l'objet d'une excision pour pouvoir créer deux orifices urétéraux dans la vessie.

Une héminéphrectomie avec excision de l'urétérocèle et réimplantation simultanée de l'urétére ipsilatéral fut pratiquée dans trois cas. Dans trois autres cas, il y avait aussi une urétérocèle importante et un reflux dans l'urétère ipsilatéral. Dans le cas d'une urétérocèle de moindre importance, sans reflux, nous avons pratiqué une néphrectomie de l'extrémité supérieure du rein et une urétérectomie partielle sans excision du moignon et de l'urétérocèle. Nous avons aussi pratiqué une excision de l'urétérocèle et une réimplantation en bloc dans un cas où les tissues rénaux étaient relativement en bon état. Les patients ont été suivis et les résultats constatés ont été satisfaisants dans la majorité des cas.

Introduction

Various surgical procedures are discussed in the treatment of double ureter and ureterocele. Our surgical management of such cases is presented here, along with our reasons for choosing the particular methods.

Patients and Methods

During the years 1973–1982, 25 patients with double ureters, including six with ureterocele, were treated at the Teheran University Children's Hospital. Distribution by age and sex is shown in Fig. 1. At the same time, 30 cases of double ureter with urinary tract infection were treated conservatively. The double ureter appeared equally frequently on each side, and in four cases it presented bilaterally. Bacteriological urine examination indicated *Escherichia coli* in the majority of the cases and *Klebsiella* in a few of them. Surgery was indicated when the urinary tract infection resisted medical treatment and when hydronephrosis appeared.

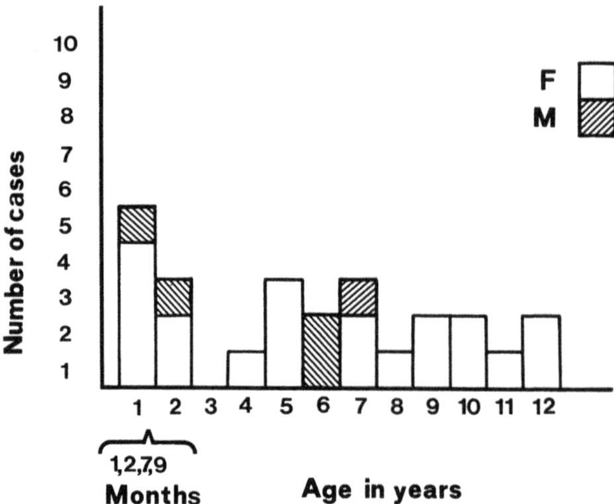

Fig. 1. Distribution of double ureter by age and sex among 25 cases from the Children's Hospital in Teheran

Table 1. Frequency of symptoms

Before 2 years of age	After 2 years of age
Fever	Dysuria
Diarrhoea	Flank pain
Failure to thrive	Fever
Abdominal mass	Enuresis
Inflamed exterior genitals	Cloudy urine
	Hypertonia

Table 2. Frequency of reflux

Vesicoureteral reflux	$n = 17$
In lower ureter	13
In upper ureter	1
In both ureters	3
Ureteroureteral reflux	$n = 10$
With lower bifurcation	6
With middle bifurcation	4

The frequency of various symptoms according to age is shown in Table 1. Table 2 shows the frequency of reflux among our 25 cases, and Table 3 gives the surgical prcoedures performed.

Case Reports

An 8-year-old girl presented with recurrent urinary tract infection and right renal colic. An excretory urogram (Fig. 2) showed uretero-ureteral reflux with incomplete ureteral duplication. An interpelvic anastomosis was performed on the right side. The results were satisfactory. Urinary infection appeared again 6 years later, but this time the renal colic was observed on the left side. Low bifurcation of the ureter was found on the left. The 3-cm-long common segment was resected and an en bloc reimplantation was performed.

A blind-ending branch of a bifid ureter was found lying prevesically on the right side in a 7-year-old girl (Fig. 3). We performed a resection and reimplantation of the ureter. The blind-ending branch was 4 cm long and 7 mm wide.

Table 3. Surgical procedures used for correction of double ureter

Procedure	Number of patients
Heminephroureterectomy	8
Upper segment − combined with excision of ureterocele in three	5
Lower segment	3
Ureteral reimplantation	6
In three cases reimplantation of ipsilateral ureter after excision of ureterocele	
En bloc reimplantation with vesicoureteral reflux UCNST "en bloc", type I	4
En bloc reimplantation with vesico-ureteral reflux in both ureters UCNST "en bloc", type II	3
En bloc reimplantation with lower bifurcation and uretero-ureteral reflux UCNST "en bloc", type III	3
Interpelvic anastomosis	2
Primary nephrectomy, both segments	1
Secondary nephrectomy, previous heminephrectomy	1
Pyelolithotomy	3

UCNST = uretero-cysto-neostomy

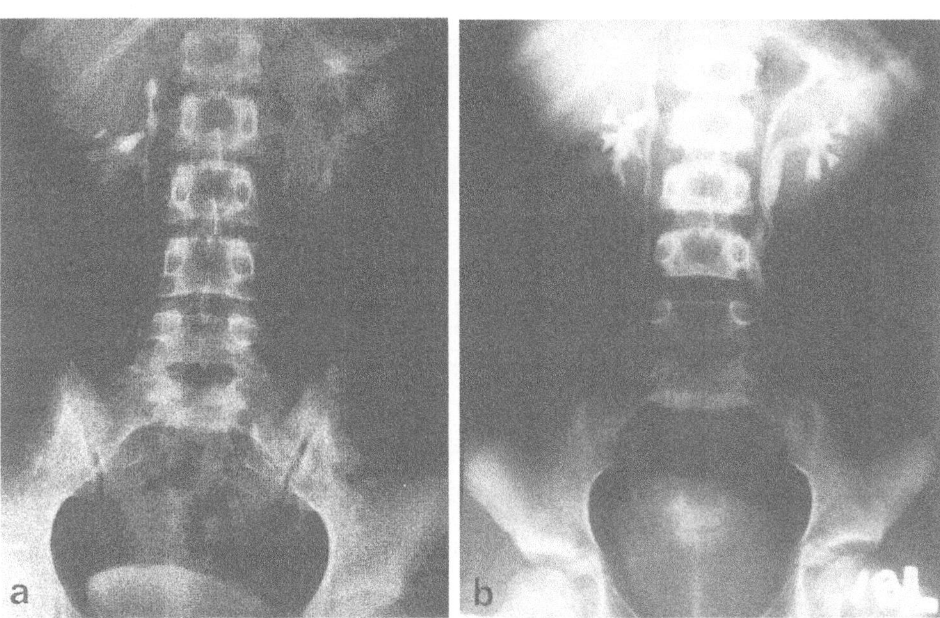

Fig. 2. a Excretory urogram in an 8-year-old girl showing uretero-ureteral reflux with incomplete ureteral duplication. On the right side the bifurcation is located in the middle and on the left side it is prevesical. **b** Excretory urogram showing interpelvic anastomosis: right side after 7 years, left side 1 year after en bloc reimplantation

In a 2-month-old female infant with urosepsis, a cystogram revealed bilateral reflux in the lower pole of bilaterally duplicated kidney and ureters. An excretory urogram (Fig. 4) showed ureterocele associated with a hydronephrotic upper pole of the left kidney. We performed resection of the ureterocele, repair of the defect in the bladder wall, and en bloc reimplantation of both ureters in a single session. An en bloc reimplantation was also performed on the right side.

A 2-year-old boy presented with urosepsis and pyuria, severe hydronephrosis and hydroureter on the left side. A large ureterocele was associated with the upper pole of the right kidney, which was destroyed and not visualizable. A cystogram (Fig. 5) showed bilateral reflux, on the right side to the lower pole, which had destroyed that half of the kidney as well. Nephrectomy on the right and ureter reimplantation on the left were performed.

Discussion

In deciding on the operative treatment of double ureter, there are generally three types to differentiate (Amar and Chabra 1970; Bettex 1965; Kelalis 1976; Maier and Simonis 1969; Sigel 1971):

1. Bifid ureter with uretero-ureteral reflux.
2. Double ureter with cystoureteral reflux: In this case either both orifices lie in the bladder with reflux in the lateral ectopic ureter, usually in the lower one, or both ureters have a common ureteral orifice with reflux occurring in both.
3. Double ureter with ureterocele: The upper pole is usually hydronephrotic and dysplastic, and the lower ureter is frequently accompanied by reflux.

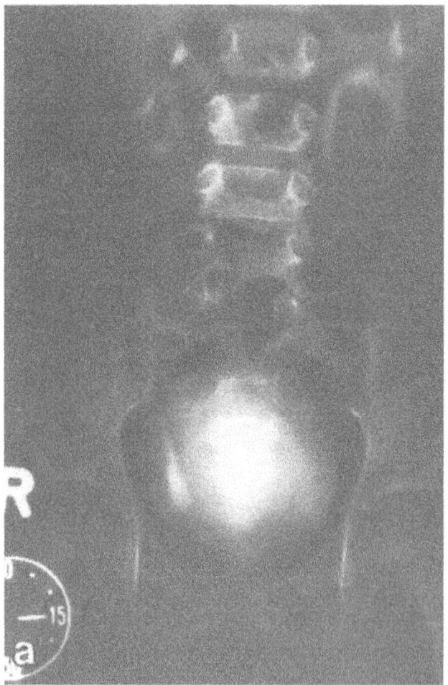

Fig. 3. a Excretory urogram in a 7-year-old girl with blind-ending branch of bifid ureter, demonstrated by hyperdensity of contrast medium as dilatation of the prevesical ureter. b Voiding cystogram shows vesicoureteral reflux on right side. Blind-ending branch of bifid ureter is visible. c Resected specimen. Blind-ending branch was 4 cm long and 7 mm wide

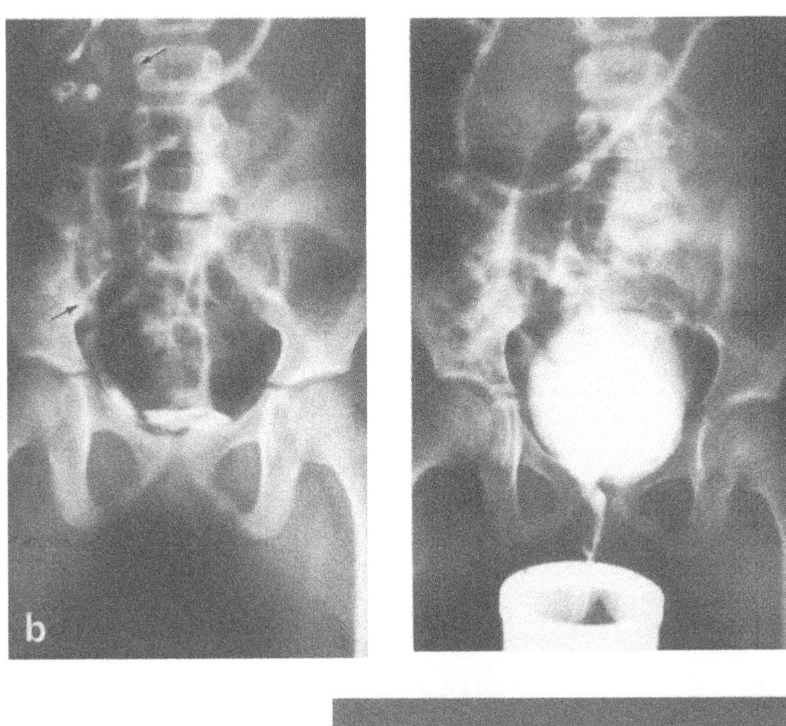

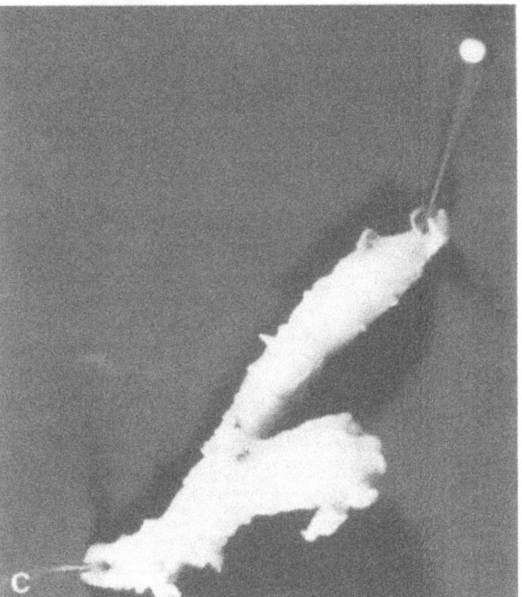

Fig. 3b, c

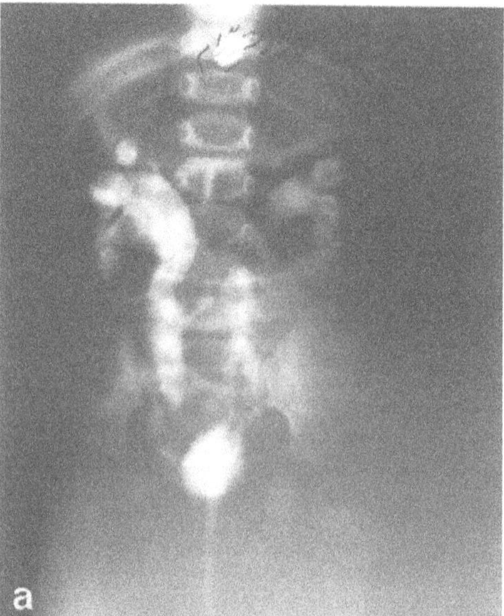

Fig. 4. a Cystogram of a 2-month-old girl, showing bilateral reflux in lower pole of bilaterally duplicated kidney and ureter. **b** Excretory urogram made 3 months after surgery

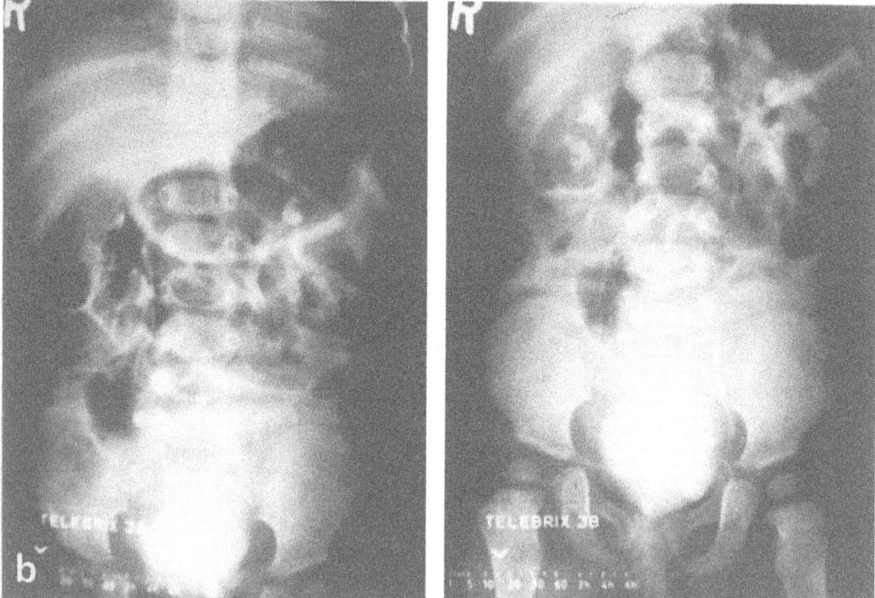

For the first group of patients we used interpelvic anastomosis after Gibson and Genton as the operative treatment (Genton 1966; Gibson 1957). Heminephrectomy was performed when the kidney was severely damaged.

En bloc reimplantation after Bettex (Bettex 1965; Bettex and Kuffer 1969) was performed as the operative treatment for the second group. In case of bifid

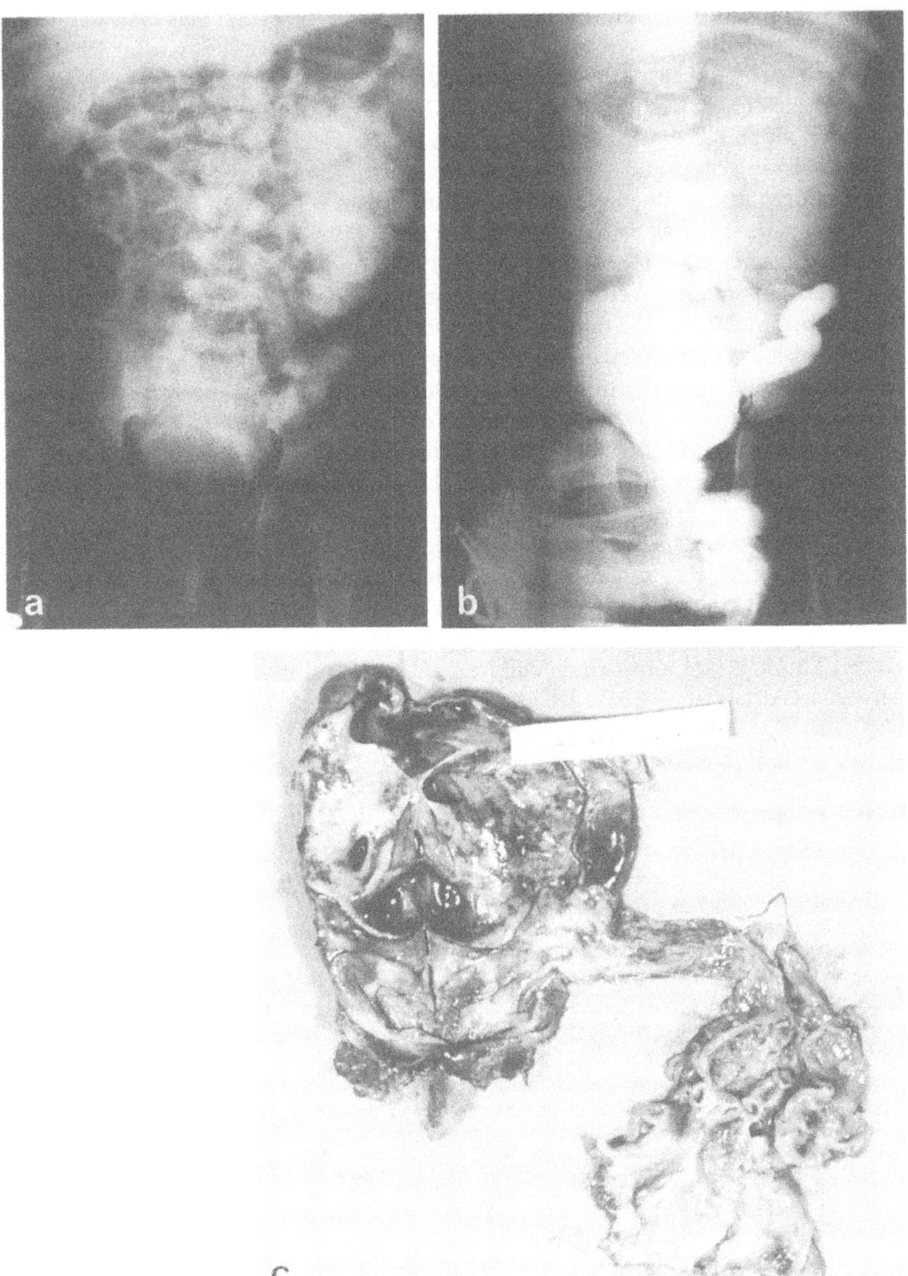

Fig. 5. a Excretory urogram in a 2-year-old boy showing large ureterocele associated with upper pole of right kidney, which is not visualized. **b** Cystogram shows bilateral reflux and displaced ureter. **c** Resected specimen: severely pyelonephrotic, atrophic kidney and severely dilated double ureter

ureter with low bifurcation, the common segment of the ureter was excised and an en bloc reimplantation was performed (Bettex 1965; Bettex and Kuffer 1969).

There is some disagreement regarding treatment of ureterocele. Hendren and Monfort (1971), Ericsson and Rhude (1957), Morger (1973) and Mildenberger et al. (1967) all prefer a radical operation with total excision of the ureterocele, heminephroureterectomy and simultaneous reimplantation of the ipsilateral ureter. They feel that the ureterocele and ureter stump are a source of infection and that the lower pole is at risk from reflux. Malek et al. (1972), Kellalis (1976), Stephens (1958), Hanson et al. (1984), Cobb et al. (1982), and Jenny and Herzog (1980) recommend heminephroureterectomy without excision of the ureterocele and ureter stump. They stress the danger of the blood supply of the ipsilateral ureter.

Our surgical preference in the treatment of large ureterocele with reflux is the radical approach. For the treatment of small ureterocele without reflux we prefer heminephroureterectomy without excision of the ureterocele and ureter stump.

Infrequently, ureteroceles with well-functioning upper poles are found. In such cases, Hendren prefers excision of the ureterocele, ureterectomy and high pyelo-pyelostomy (Hendren and Monfort 1971).

In a 2-month-old girl with a relatively well preserved upper renal pole, we performed an en bloc reimplantation with excision of the ureterocele. We prefer ureterectomy with pyelo-pyelostomy when the ureter is severely dilated.

Among our patients was a 7-year-old girl with a blind-ending branch of a bifid ureter. This is a rare anomaly in children and is found mostly in girls, and on the right side (Albers et al. 1968; Kelalis 1976; Schultze 1967).

References

Albers DD, Geyer JR, Barnes SD (1968) Blind-ending branch of bifid ureter: report of 3 cases. J Urol 99:160–164

Amar AD, Chabra K (1970) Reflux in duplicated ureters: treatment in children. J Pediatr Surg 5:419–430

Bettex M (1965) Über den vesico-ureteralen Reflux beim Säugling und Kind. Huber, Bern

Bettex M, Kuffer FR (1969) Indikationen und Ergebnisse der Uretero-cystoneostomie bei refluierenden Doppelureteren im Kindesalter. Z Kinderchir 7:489–499

Cobb M, Desai PG, Price SE (1982) Surgical management of infantile (ectopic) ureteroceles: report of a modified approach. J Pediatr Surg 17:745–748

Ericsson N, Rhude U (1957) The lower urinary tract in childhood, vol 10. Almquist & Wiksell, Stockholm, pp 114–146

Genton N (1966) L'anastomose interpyélic dans la chirurgie du double-rein. Z Kinderchir [Suppl] 101–115

Gibson TE (1957) A new operation for ureteral ectopia: case report. J Urol 77:414

Hanson E, Enger EA, Hjahnas K (1984) Heminephrectomy-ureterectomy as the sole procedure in ectopic ureterocele in children. Z Kinderchir 39:355–357

Hendren WH, Monfort GJ (1971) Surgical correction of ureteroceles in childhood. J Pediatr Surg 6:235–244

Jenny P, Herzog B (1982) Zur Therapie der Ureterocele. Z Kinderchir 35:106–108

Kelalis PP (1976) Anomalies of the urinary tract, renal pelvis and ureter. In: Kelalis PP, Kiney LR, Belman AB (eds) Clinical pediatric urology, vol 1. Saunders, Philadelphia, pp 503–541

Maier WA, Simonis P (1969) Erfahrungen in der chirurgischen Behandlung von Nierendoppelungen mit Doppelureter. Z Kinderchir 7:477–488

Malek RS, Kelalis PP, Burke EC, Strickler GB (1972) Simple and ectopic ureterocele in infancy and childhood. Surg Gynecol Obstet 134:611–616

Mildenberger H, Flach A, Fendel H (1967) Die Behandlung der Ureterocele im Kindesalter. Z Kinderchir 4:204–210

Morger R (1973) Beitrag zur Ureterocele beim Kind. Z Kinderchir 13:234–240

Schultze R (1967) Der blindendende Doppelureter. Z Urol Nephrol 60:271–289

Sigel A (1971) Doppelniere und Doppelharnleiter. Lehrbuch der Kinderurologie. Thieme, Stuttgart, pp 250–277

Stephens FD (1958) Ureterocele in infants and children. Aust NZ J Surg 27:288–295

Surgical Treatment of Bilateral Wilms' Tumours with Special Reference to Second Operations in Metachronous Disease

W. Pumberger and P. Wurnig

Summary

We report on six patients with bilateral Wilms' tumours (among them one pair of siblings) who underwent surgery within a period of 20 years. Wilms' tumours appeared synchronously in three patients and successively in the other three. Case reports are given for three of the six patients. The tumours have a remarkable multilocular appearance, indicating a multilocular genesis. In this context, the phenomenon of nephroblastomatosis is discussed. In addition to surgical treatment, aggressive conservative therapy should be employed, particularly with metachronous disease and the resulting acquired solitary kidney in these patients.

Zusammenfassung

Es wird über die chirurgische Therapie bei 6 Patienten mit bilateralen Wilms-Tumoren berichtet (davon 1 Geschwisterpaar). Der Beobachtungszeitraum erstreckt sich über 20 Jahre. Bei 3 Kindern wurde der Tumor synchron, bei 3 Kindern nacheinander diagnostiziert. Drei dieser Patienten werden gesondert vorgestellt. Auffällig ist das gehäuft multilokuläre Vorkommen der Tumoren, welches auf eine multilokuläre Tumorgenese schließen läßt. In diesem Zusammenhang wird auf das Phänomen der Nephroblastomatose eingegangen. Zusätzlich zur chirurgischen Therapie bietet sich besonders bei metachronem Verlauf und der dadurch bedingten Einnierigkeit ein konservativ aggressives Vorgehen als Therapie der Wahl an.

Résumé

Il est fait état du traitement chirurgical de 6 patients atteints de tumeurs de Wilms bilatérales (dont deux enfants de la même fratrie). Ces patients ont été suivis pendant 20 ans. Trois enfants présentaient les deux tumeurs dès l'abord alors que les trois autres les ont présentées successivement. Trois de ces cas sont détaillés ici. On notera l'apparition fréquente de tumeurs multiloculaires qui indiqueraient une genèse multiloculaire. Dans ce contexte, on traite ensuite de la néphroblastomatose.

Dept. Paed. Surgery, Mautner Markhofsches Kinderspital of Vienna, Baumgasse 75, A-1030 Vienna, Austria

Progress in Pediatric Surgery, Vol. 23
Ed. by L. Spitz et al.
© Springer-Verlag Berlin Heidelberg 1989

Il semble alors que la thérapeutique de choix soit, outre le traitement chirurgical, une thérapeutique conservatrice agressive, surtout dans le cas de l'apparition successive des tumeurs et du rein unique qui en résulterait.

Whereas the treatment of unilateral stage I–IV Wilms' tumours is to a large extent standardized and yields good results (Gutjahr 1981), no general rules of therapy for bilateral Wilms' tumours (stage V) exist. In stage V, there is bilateral affection of the kidneys, either synchronous or metachronous. Four percent to eleven percent of all Wilms' tumours are stage V, and 67% of patients are less than 2 years of age. There is a slight prevalence of male patients, familial appearance is not uncommon, and the genesis is frequently multilocular. Owing to the special characteristics of this group of patients, surgical treatment must be adapted to the individual situation (Lago et al. 1985; Ragab et al. 1972; White et al. 1976). The individuality of each case increases over the longterm due to changes and further developments in surgery, radiology and chemotherapy.

Patients

From 1965 to 1985, six children with bilateral Wilms' tumours underwent surgery at the Mautner Markhof Children's Hospital of Vienna (Table 1). Tumours were diagnosed simultaneously in three children (cases 1–3, Table 1), although therapy ensued successively in case 3 (preceding unilateral nephrectomy performed in

Table 1. Bilateral Wilms' tumours (1965–1985), clinical data

Patient	Age at time of diagnosis I	Interval to diagnosis II	Multi-locular appear-ance	Course
Simultaneous				
1) S.P., female, no. 15482/83	4 years and 4 months	–	–	Died of generalized metastases
2) S.I., female[a], no. 15422/83	8 months	–	+	At present (3 years) free of recurrence
3) H.M., male,	4 years and	1 month	+	Unknown
Subsequent				
4) R.D., male, no. 11595/65	1.5 years	3 years and 4 months	–	Cured (20 years)
5) M.H., male, no. 11596/73	5 months	11 months	–	Died 3 months later
6) F.I., male[a], no. 5408/73	4 months	14 months	+	Cured (13 years)

[a] Siblings

another hospital). In three children diagnosis was made successively (cases 4–6), whereby the longest time interval was 3 years, 4 months. In four cases the tumours were discovered before the second year of life. Among our six patients were a pair of siblings in whom diagnosis was made in the first year of life (cases 2 and 6). Three cases will be described individually below.

Case Reports

Case 6. F.I., male, no. 5408/1973. The patient was diagnosed as having a tumour in the right upper abdomen on the occasion of a herniorrhaphy at the age of 4 months. A right-sided tumour nephrectomy was carried out, revealing multilocular invasion of the kidney with two separate tumour nodes (3 and 5 cm in diameter). Histology showed a mixed-type nephroblastoma.

Postoperatively, the boy was given actinomycin D but no irradiation. He presented 14 months later with a fist-sized tumour in the left medium abdomen. An i.v. pyelogram showed compression of the left renal cavity from above and below. Preoperative chemotherapy (actinomycin D) and irradiation effected considerable tumour reduction. Intraoperatively, two apple-sized tumours at the upper and lower pole were enucleated, the lower by complete enucleation and suturing of the tumour bed, the upper only by morcellation (Fig. 1a, b). Chemotherapy and irradiation were continued (up to 2000 rads) postoperatively.

Today, the patient, aged 13 years, is free of complaints and has normal renal parameters as well as good renal function as seen on the i.v. pyelogram (Fig. 1c). A review of roentgenograms disclosed a slight, scarcely recognizable change at the upper renal cavity at the time of the first operation; this was, however, not palpable, and ultrasonography was not yet available.

Case 1. S.P., female, 4 yrs, no. 15482/1983. An i.v. pyelogram disclosed the typical picture of a Wilms' tumour, which was clearly palpable in the right upper abdomen, whereas only a slight impression of the left upper renal cavity could be seen (Fig. 2a). Palpation findings on the left side were normal preoperatively. Ultrasonography revealed a tumour 2.5 cm in diameter within the left upper renal pole (Fig. 2b). These findings were confirmed on laparotomy; a tumour nephrectomy was carried out on the right side, as was a tangential resection of the IVC for tumour invasion of the renal vein at the junction with the IVC. The tumour on the left side was enucleated from the upper pole. Histology showed a blastomatous tumour with marked anaplasia. The girl died of generalized metastases a few months later. It should be noted that tumours with vessel invasion tend toward diffuse metastasis.

Case 3. H.M., male, 4.5 yrs, no. 20825/1984. This boy was nephrectomized because of a left-sided Wilms' tumour in July 1984. At that time tumorous changes at the right upper renal pole were suspected. The boy was transferred to us 1

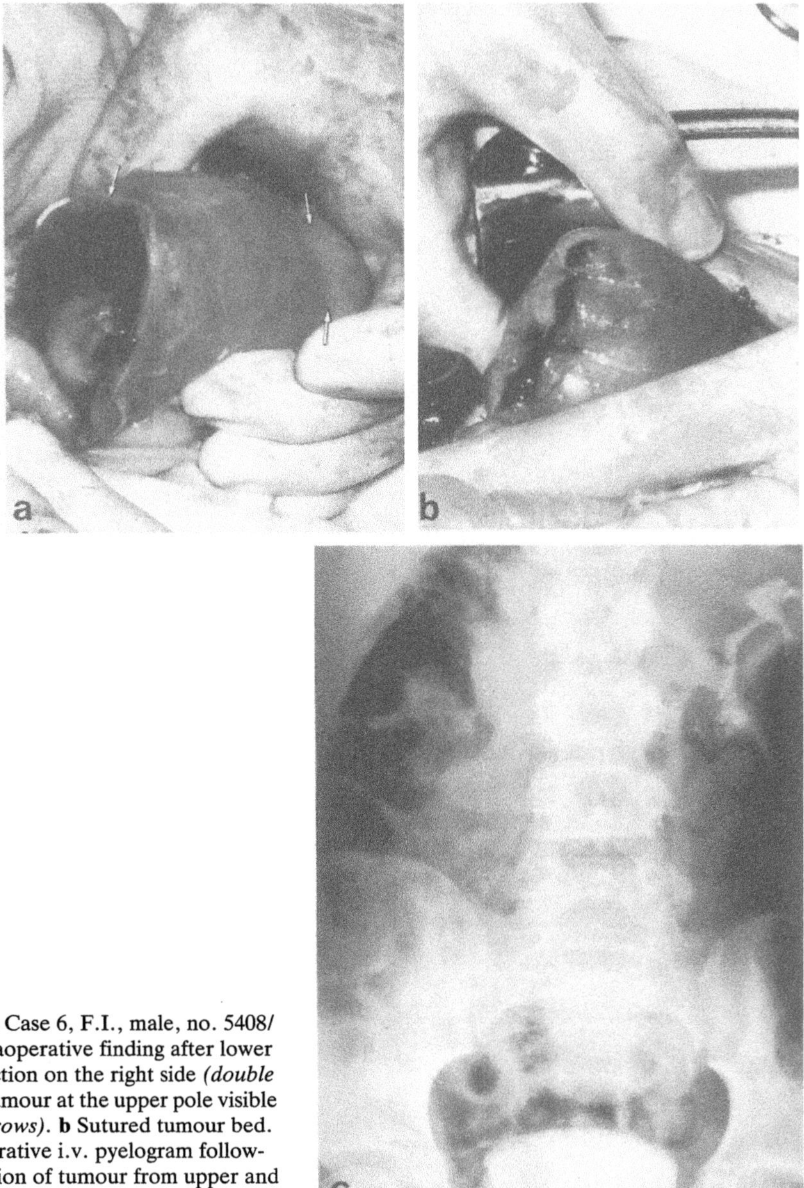

Fig. 1a–c. Case 6, F.I., male, no. 5408/
73. **a** Intraoperative finding after lower
pole resection on the right side *(double
arrow);* tumour at the upper pole visible
(single arrows). **b** Sutured tumour bed.
c Postoperative i.v. pyelogram following resection of tumour from upper and
lower renal poles

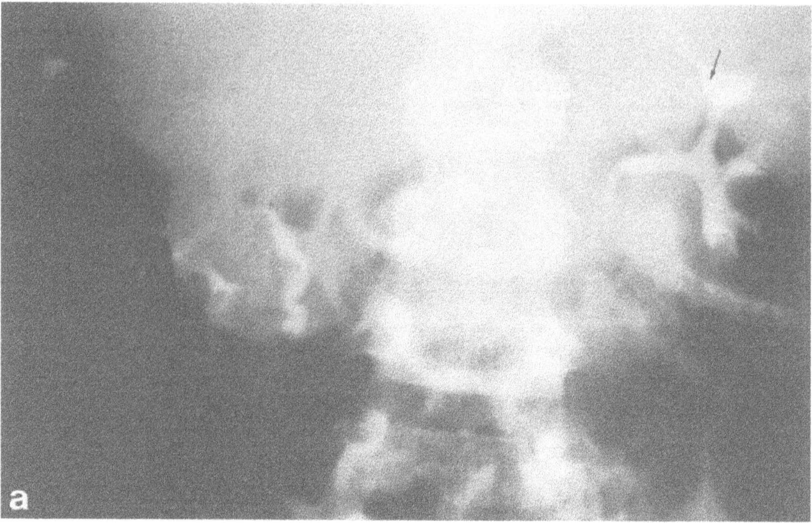

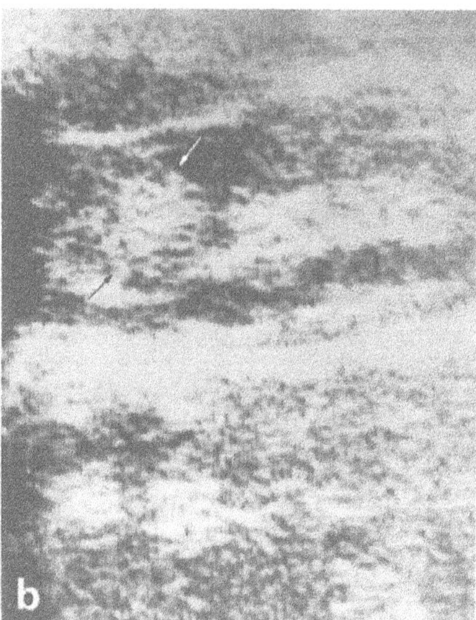

Fig. 2a, b. Case 1, S.P., female, no. 15482/83.
a Preoperative i.v. pyelogram: *right,* typical deformation by Wilms tumour; *left,* slight impression of the upper calices *(arrow).* Left tumour could not be palpated preoperatively.
b Ultrasound picture of the left kidney: tumour node 2.5 cm in diameter at the upper pole *(arrows)*

month later. Despite irradiation and chemotherapy, the tumour showed significant progression. On laparotomy, three separate tumor nodes were found in the right kidney (one fist-sized node at the upper pole, one 5 cm in diameter at the lower pole and a smaller node in the middle of the kidney). The nodes were excised by diathermy while the kidney was hypoperfused by clamping of the renal vessels for 30 min (Fig. 3a, b). There was good perfusion of the kidney after the operation, and an i.v. pyelogram showed good renal function. Histology revealed blastomatous-type Wilms' tumours without anaplasia in all three nodes. The further course cannot be assessed since the boy lives far away.[1]

Discussion

Both in the literature (Heidemann et al. 1975; Lago et al. 1985) and among our patients, there is a notable frequency of multilocular tumours. In five kidneys in three children (cases 2, 3 and 6) discrete multilocular tumours were found. In the context of multilocular affection, the phenomenon of nephroblastomatosis seems to be of great importance (Heidemann et al. 1975); it is found in 30%–40% of all patients with Wilms' tumours. Nephroblastomatosis involves bilateral, multilocular changes of renal tissue on the basis of embryonic tissue (Bove and McAdams 1976). It can present as a nodular renal blastema (i.e. a nephroblastoma in situ), as a metanephric hamartoma, or as a small monomorphic Wilms' tumour 1–3.5 cm in diameter. Its practical significance lies in its potential premalignancy and in its indication of bilateral occurrence (the familial appearance in siblings is very remarkable).

If nephroblastomatosis is detected in a Wilms' tumour of an excised kidney, it can be an important hint at the existence of a second Wilms' tumour. Excised kidneys bearing Wilms' tumour should be examined histologically for nephroblastomatous changes in their non-tumorous regions. There are various choices of surgical therapy for bilateral Wilms' tumours; in metachronous disease a unilateral nephrectomy has already been carried out:

1. Bilateral tumor enucleation (Wiener 1976), almost always applicable if the diagnosis is made simultaneously
2. Unilateral nephrectomy and contralateral heminephrectomy (mostly in metachronous disease if tumour nephrectomy has already been performed). Contralateral heminephrectomy can be modified as follows: tumour excision by diathermy, cryosurgery or laser under temporary ischaemia (hypoperfusion)
3. Extracorporeal (cryosurgical) tumor excision and autotransplantation (bench surgery; Anderson and Altman 1976; Lilly et al. 1975)
4. Uni- or bilateral renal transplantation, possible with both simultaneous and successive diagnosis

Unilateral tumour nephrectomy had already been performed in all of our patients with metachronous disease. When the tumour on the contralateral side was diagnosed in one case it was found to be inoperable, and the parents did not consent to excision of the remaining kidney. In one other case a heminephrectomy was carried out.

---

[1]Pathohistology courtesy of Prof. Dr. Krepler, Pathological Institute (Dir., Prof. Dr. Holzner) of the University of Vienna

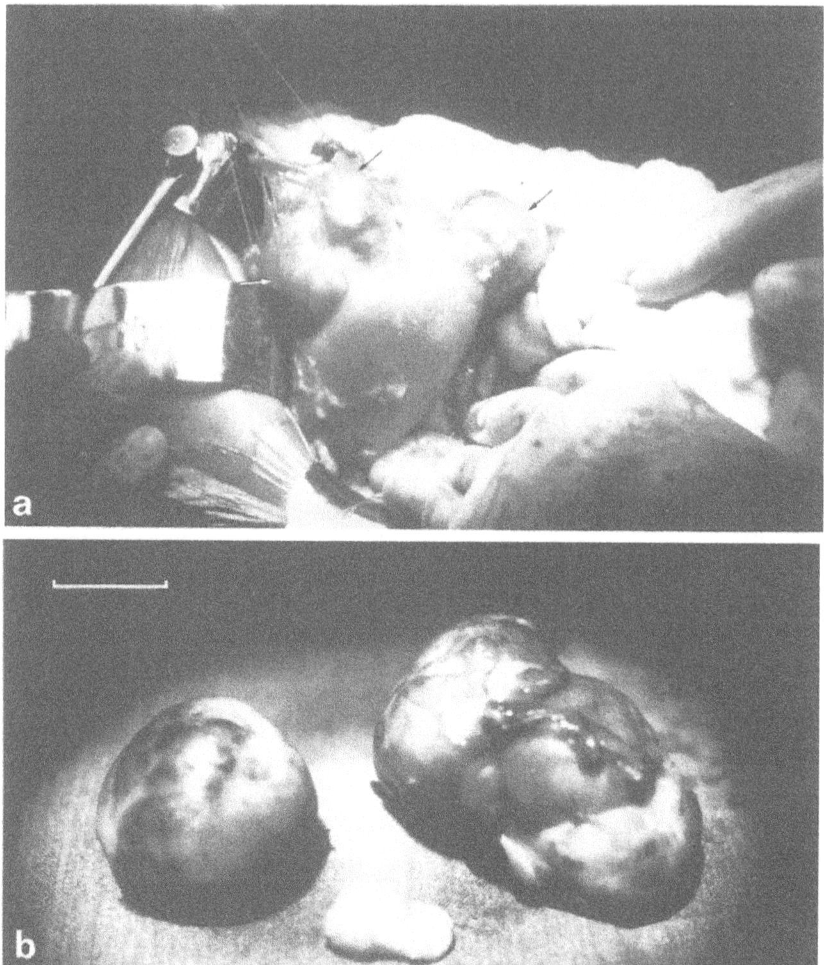

Fig. 3a, b. Case 3, H.M., male, no. 20825/84. State after tumour nephrectomy on the left side, subsequent operation on the right. **a** Intraoperative situs, multilocular nodes *(arrows)*. **b** Three tumour nodes removed from the right kidney. *Bar* = 2 cm

Before ultrasonography and computer tomography became available, bilateral appearance was not diagnosed in 30% of cases. Table 2 gives our surgical procedures in cases of synchronous disease.

Young age, multilocular occurrence and a possible metachronous course require exact consideration of the individual situation. Despite advancements in surgical techniques (Anderson and Altman 1976; Lilly et al. 1975; deMaria et al. 1979), conservative surgical procedures seem to be the methods of choice even today (Lago et al. 1985; Ragab et al. 1972; White et al. 1976; Wiener 1976). This

Table 2. Surgical treatment in cases of synchronous appearance

1. S.P., female, no. 15482/83	Right side Left side	Tumour nephrectomy and tangential resection of IVC Tumour enucleation
2. S.I., female, no. 15422/83	Right side Left side	Tumour nephrectomy Lower pole resection and enucleation of a second, smaller node
3. H.M., male, no. 20825/84	Left side Right side	Tumour nephrectomy Enucleation of three nodes of different sizes under hypoperfusion for 30 min

does not necessarily mean that radical excision of the tumour at any price is required (Bishop et al. 1977); subsequent to surgery, irradiation and chemotherapy can be applied with good results in stage I–IV Wilms' tumours.

References

Anderson KD, Altman RP (1976) Selective resection of malignant tumors using bench surgical techniques. J Pediatr Surg 11:881–882

Bishop HC, Tefft M, Evans AE, D'Angio GJ (1977) Survival in bilateral Wilms' tumor – review of 30 national Wilms'-tumor study cases. J Pediatr Surg 12:631–638

Bove KE, McAdams AJ (1976) The nephroblastomosis complex and its relationship to Wilms' tumour: a clinicopathologic treatise. Perspect Pediatr Pathol 3:185

deMaria JE, Hardy BE, Brezinski A, Churchill BM (1979) Renal transplantation in patients with bilateral Wilms' tumor. J Pediatr Surg 14:577–579

Gutjahr P (1981) Ergebnisse der Behandlung von Wilms-Tumoren nach einem Plan (I/76) der Gesellschaft für Pädiatrische Onkologie – eine retrospektive Analyse. Ergeb Padiatr Onkol 5:119–135

Heidemann RL, Haase GM, Foley CL, Wilson HL, Bailey WC (1975) Nephroblastomatosis and Wilms' tumor. Cancer 55:1446–1451

Lago CM, Gonzalez FC, Lorenzo CG, López-Pérez (1985) Bilateral multifocal Wilms' tumor. J Pediatr Surg 20:552–553

Lilly JR, Pfister RR, Putnam CW, Kosloske AM, Starzl TE (1975) Bench surgery and renal autotransplantation in the pediatric patient. J Pediatr Surg 10:623–630

Ragab AH, Vietti TJ, Crist W, Perez C, McAllister W (1972) Bilateral Wilms' tumor, a review. Cancer 30:983–998

White JJ, Golladay ES, Kaizer H, Pinney JD, Haller JA (1976) Conservatively agressive management with bilateral Wilms' tumors. J Pediatr Surg 11:859–865

Wiener ES (1976) Bilateral partial nephrectomies for large bilateral Wilms' tumors. J Pediatr Surg 11:867–869

Infants with Posterior Urethral Valves:
A Retrospective Study and Consequences for Therapy

H. Mildenberger, R. Habenicht, and H. Zimmermann

Summary

This is a report on the follow-up data of 18 patients with posterior urethral valves diagnosed during the first year of life. One infant died of progressive renal failure; a slight elevation of serum creatinine levels in three children aged 4–6 years indicated a doubtful prognosis. On initial examination, ten patients showed severe unilateral or bilateral reflux. Seven of 14 refluxing units remained non-functioning and had to be removed. Following transurethral fulguration of the valves, five infants developed unilateral or bilateral reflux which was not evident on initial preoperative voiding cystograms. In contrast to those in other series, none of these refluxes ceased spontaneously. Ureteral reimplantations were done on 11 ureters of eight patients, but regression of ureteral dilatation postoperatively remained unsatisfactory in six instances, none of whom had a true mechanical obstruction. We conclude that many of these megaloureters encountered in infants with posterior urethral valves are concomitant with profound and often irreversible damage of the ureter wall. Surgery of such ureters, therefore, should be avoided whenever feasible.

Zusammenfassung

Es wird eine katamnestische Untersuchung über 18 Patienten mit posterioren Urethralklappen vorgelegt, bei denen diese Diagnose bereits im Neugeborenen- oder Säuglingsalter gestellt worden war. Eines der Kinder verstarb an progredientem Nierenversagen, während bei 3 Kindern eine leichte Erhöhung des Serumkreatininwertes eine zweifelhafte Prognose erkennen ließ. Zehn der Kinder zeigten bereits bei der initialen MCU-Untersuchung einen massiven ein- oder beidseitigen Reflux. Sieben der 14 refluxiven Ureter-Niereneinheiten blieben funktionslos und mußten entfernt werden. Nach der transurethralen Elektrofulguration der Klappen trat bei 5 Säuglingen ein- oder beidseitig ein Reflux auf, der bei der Primäruntersuchung noch nicht nachweisbar war. Im Gegensatz zu den Beobachtungen anderer Autoren, verschwand während der Beobachtungszeit kein Reflux spontan. Bei 8 Patienten wurden 11 Ureter neu in die Blase implantiert. Jedoch blieb der Rückgang der Ureterdilatation postoperativ bei 6 dieser Ureter ungenü-

Kinderchirurgische Abteilung, Medizinische Hochschule Hannover, Federal Republic of Germany

Progress in Pediatric Surgery, Vol. 23
Ed. by L. Spitz et al.
© Springer-Verlag Berlin Heidelberg 1989

gend, obgleich eine mechanische Obstruktion in keinem Fall nachgewiesen werden konnte. Wir schließen daraus, daß bei vielen dieser mit posterioren Urethralklappen vergesellschafteten Megauretern eine tiefgreifende und oftmals irreversible Schädigung der Ureterwandstruktur vorliegt. Operationen an diesen Uretern sollten deshalb soweit als nur möglich vermieden werden.

Résumé

Il s'agit d'une étude des données obtenues en suivant 18 patients porteurs de valves urétrales postérieures, le diagnostic ayant été posé quand les patients étaient nouveaux-nés ou nourrissons. Un des enfants est décédé l'une néphroparalysie et dans le cas de trois autres, âgés de 4 à 6 ans, une légère élévation du taux de créatinine plasmatique assombrit le pronostic. Quand ils furent examinés pour la première fois, 10 des patients présentaient un reflux grave unilatéral ou bilatéral. 7 reins avec reflux sur 14 continuèrent à ne pas fonctionner et durent faire l'objet d'une ablation. Après électrofulguration transurétrale des valves, un reflux unilatéral ou bilatéral apparut dans le cas de 5 nourrissons ce qui n'était pas décelable lors du premier examen. Contrairement aux observations rapportées par d'autres auteurs, aucun reflux n'a disparu spontanément. Dans le cas de 8 patients, 11 uretères ont été implantés dans la vessie.

Dans six cas, la réduction post-opératoire de la dilatation de l'uretère ne fut pas suffisante et ce, malgré l'absence de toute obstruction mécanique. Nous en concluons que dans beaucoup de ces méga-uretères associés à des valves urétrales postérieures, il s'est produit une lésion souvent irréversible de la structure pariétale de l'uretère.

Il faut donc autant que possible éviter de pratiquer des interventions sur ces uretères.

A high rate of complications and failures in the surgical treatment of ureters in infants suffering from posterior urethral valves (Atwell 1983; Bachman et al. 1985) requires a restrictive indication for operative corrections (Evins and Lorenzo 1979; Saalfield et al. 1976). We hereby report our experience in applying such a restrictive strategy in our patients during the period from 1978 to 1984.

Patients

The study group consisted of 18 patients who presented during the first year of life, predominantly during the neonatal period. At hospital admission 11 patients were less than 1 week old, two were 2 and 4 weeks old, respectively, and five presented between 1 and 12 months of age.

Presenting signs of study patients are listed in Table 1. In five cases the main symptom was a "tumour" in the lower abdomen, usually associated with urinary retention and/or a poor urinary stream. In eight cases urinary tract infection, in-

Table 1. Presenting sign in 18 infants with posterior urethral valves

Bladder tumour	5
Septicaemia, renal failure	5
Urinary tract infection	3
Bilateral pneumothoraces	1
Prenatal diagnosis	3
Accidental finding at abdominal ultrasonography	1

Table 2. Creatinine determination on admission (µmol/l)

	No. of patients
Below 60	7
60 – 99	3
100 – 199	3
200 and more	5

Table 3. Frequency of reflux in 18 infants

Unilateral	
– left	3
– right	3
Bilateral	4

cluding five cases of septicaemia and azotaemia, was the presenting symptom. The diagnosis of posterior urethral valves had been suspected on prenatal ultrasonography in three cases. One newborn with respiratory distress was found to have bilateral pneumothoraces, a not unusual finding in newborns with urethral valves (Nakayama 1986).

Normal renal function was found in seven infants (Table 2). In contrast, there was a significant impairment of renal function as assessed by increased serum creatinine in five patients. One of the infants in this subgroup died of progressive renal failure at the age of 3 months.

Severe unilateral vesicoureteral reflux was found on initial voiding cystography in six infants, and four patients were found to have bilateral reflux (Table 3). The kidneys in five of six patients with unilateral reflux were nonfunctioning, and they did not regain any function after operative diversion. These five kidneys were ultimately removed. One of the unilateral refluxes occurred into a ruptured kidney with a large perirenal extravasation (Fig. 1): this kidney was found to take up function almost immediately after bladder drainage. Four of the five nephrectomized children showed normal kidney function according to their creatinine level (below 70 µmol/l) and a normal renal iodohippurate sodium I 123 scintiscan at follow-up 1–6 years after operation. One patient, however, was found to have a creatinine level of 101 µmol/l and an impairment of his creatinine clearance to 45 ml/min/1.73 m^2 at the age of 6 years. Therefore, his prognosis regarding renal function seems doubtful (Warshaw et al. 1985).

Two of four patients presenting with bilateral refluxing ureters on initial examination each had one nonfunctioning kidney, and nephrectomy had to be per-

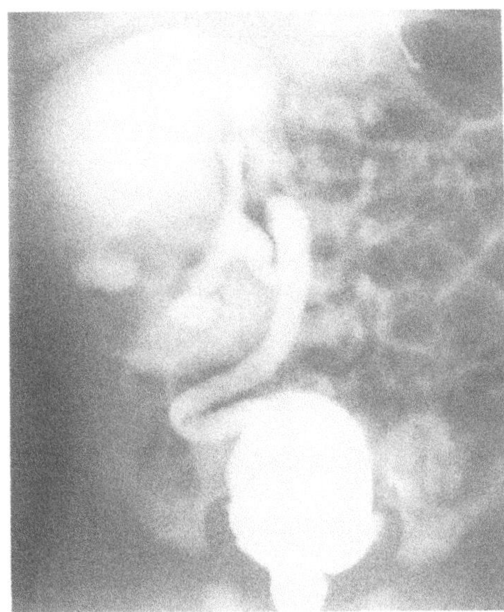

Fig. 1. Spontaneous rupture of right kidney; extensive perirenal extravasation

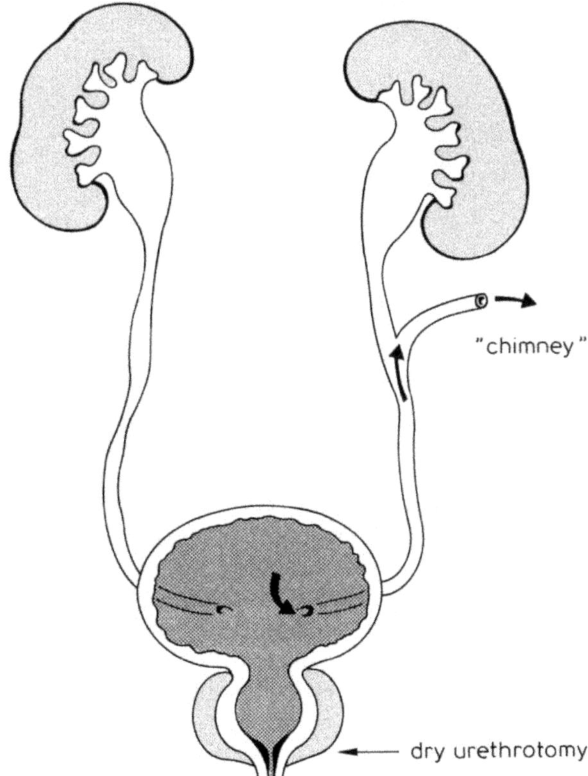

Fig. 2. Bladder evacuation via refluxing ureter and "chimney" ureterostomy, resulting in a dry urethrotomy

Table 4. Indications for ureteral reimplantation in eight patients

Dry urethrotomy	3
Severe persisting reflux	4
Obstructive bladder diverticulum	1

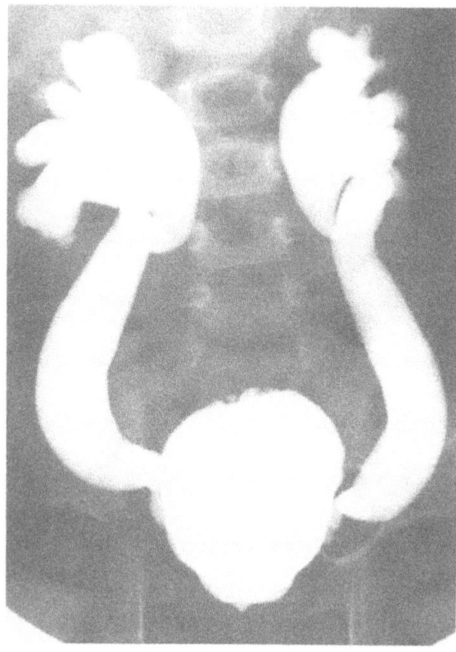

Fig. 3. Severe bilateral reflux despite prolonged bladder drainage

formed. Both of these show a low-degree renal insufficiency (creatinine 90 μmol/l and 130 μmol/l respectively) at the age of 4 years. The other two are presently in good health; one, however, has a reduced global renal function to about two thirds of normal values, as measured by renal scan.

Another observation in respect of reflux deserves mention. It was our intention to remove the urethral obstruction early in the course of treatment, and thereby to achieve early functional training of the bladder. Following transurethral fulguration of the valves, a reflux was found in five infants which had not been observed on initial examination. These new refluxes occurred in about every third ureter which had not been refluxing previously. If we take into account the fact that some of these patients had a "chimney ureterostomy" for renal protection, these new refluxes effected a bladder evacuation via refluxing ureter and ureterostomy (Fig. 2), resulting in a "dry urethrotomy". This, in turn, was accompanied by the danger of a urethral stricture (Crooks 1982), and, indeed, we saw one almost complete urethral occlusion. We therefore did a reflux-preventing ureteral

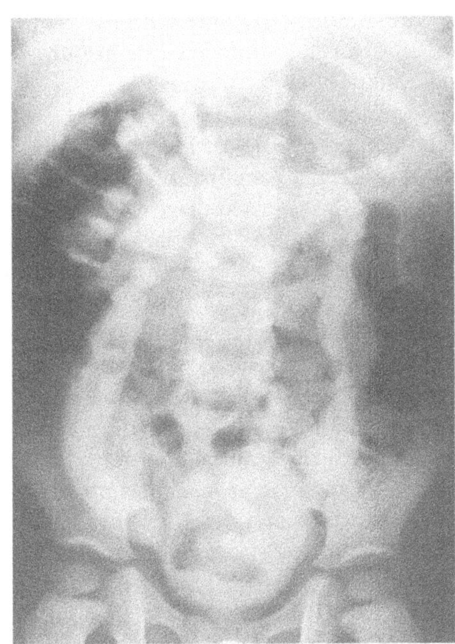

Fig. 4. Massively dilated ureters 6 months after ureteral reimplantation; same case as in Fig. 3

Table 5. Surgical strategy followed in 18 patients

	Number of patients	Prognosis		
		Good	Doubt-ful	Died
Valve fulguration only with/without ureterostomy	7	6		1
Valve fulguration with/without ureterostomy plus nephrectomy	3	2	1	
Valve fulguration plus unilateral ureteral reimplantation	1	1		
Valve fulguration with/without ureterostomy plus bilateral ureteral reimplantation	3	3		
Valve fulguration with/without ureterostomy plus nephrectomy, plus ureteral reimplantation	4	2	2	

reimplantation, together with the reopening of the urethra. In this and two other infants, a reflux-induced dry urethrostomy served as an indication for ureteral reimplantation.

The last point to be mentioned is the evaluation of ureters which need to be reimplanted (Table 4). In our patients none of these severe refluxes ceased spontaneously during an observation period of between 12 and 21 months. Therefore, six ureters in four children were reimplanted for persisting reflux. In one case, a reimplant was done for a large obstructing bladder diverticulum.

At follow-up examinations, three of 11 reimplanted ureters showed severe dilatation, suggestive of a mechanical obstruction. Operative revision of these ureters was done, but no obstruction was detected. Three other ureters exhibited moderate postoperative dilatation; four regained a normal shape. One ureter still showed reflux after surgery.

The voiding cystography of one of our patients at the age of 21 months is depicted in Fig. 3. Despite long-term bladder draining by cystostomy during the preceding 12 months, severe bilateral reflux persisted, and a ureteral reimplantation was done. Six months after the operation, an i.v. pyelogram revealed massive dilatation of both ureters (Fig. 4). No mechanical obstruction was found at re-exploration.

Finally, Table 5 presents a summary of the surgical interventions undertaken in all our infant patients with posterior urethral valves.

Discussion

In planning the operative treatment for our 18 infants with posterior urethral valves, the declared intention was to remain as conservative as possible and in particular to avoid ureteral reimplantations, as these operations are known to carry a high risk of failure (Atwell 1983; Bachmann et al. 1985). The follow-up data presented here, however, clearly indicate that this goal was not achieved.

Seven of 18 patients had to undergo nephrectomy for a non-functioning kidney. Reflux on initial examination evidently represents a grave prognostic sign (Greenfield et al. 1983) regarding kidney function: 50% of the kidneys associated with massive reflux did not regain any function following a high diversion, another 20% recovered to a limited extent only. Fairly good function, however, was found in the case of a spontaneous kidney rupture. Thus, this case may be taken as an argument in favour of the protective effect of such an event upon the involved kidney (Adzik et al. 1985; Greenfield et al. 1982).

In contrast to the experience of other authors (Egani and Smith; Kurth et al. 1981; Vaage et al. 1974), we saw no spontaneous regression of severe refluxes in our own patients. This is probably due to the stratification of our case material, restricted to newborns and infants, i.e. an age-group which shows the most serious sequelae of obstructive uropathy, among which damage to the ureterovesical junction is often irreversible.

Atwell (1983) reported a complication rate of nearly 50% following refashioning and reimplantation of ureters, caused by "poor draining of the upper tract." In our own group of patients, regression of ureteral dilatation following ureteral reimplant was unsatisfactory in more than half of the cases. Ureteral motility, probably, was equally compromised in these cases. We did not see progressive ureteral dilatations postoperatively, but rather a slow improvement over months and years. Still, this is in marked contrast to the almost invariably good results of ureteral reimplantion done on primary megaloureters without urethral valves.

The data indicate that there must be profound damage to the microstructure of the ureter wall, which proves to be irreversible in some cases of posterior urethral valves (Hanna et al. 1977). It is not clear at present whether or not such structural damage signalizes a strict contraindication for ureteral reimplants, even in cases of severe persisting reflux (Bachmann et al. 1985).

In severely impaired infants with posterior urethral valves, a percutaneous nephrostomy or a high "chimney" ureterostomy serves as an effective way to decompress the obstructed kidney (Egami and Smith 1982; Evins and Lorenzo 1979; Saalfield et al. 1976). Both methods, however, are prone to result in a "dry urethrotomy" following fulguration of the valves, if there is an accompanying refluxing ureter (Crooks 1982; Myers and Walker 1981). Our follow-up data suggest that it may be better strategy in most cases to do a vesicostomy (Egami and Smith 1982; Zaontz 1984) without direct decompression of the kidney and, in case of reflux, to postpone fulguration of the valves.

References

Adzick NS, Harrison MR, Flake AW, de Lorimier AA (1985) Urinary extravasation in the fetus with obstructive uropathy. J Pediatr Surg 20:608–615

Atwell JD (1983) Posterior urethral valves in the British Isles: a multicenter B.A.P.S. review. J Pediatr Surg 18:70–74

Bachmann H, Behrendt H, Pistor K, Olbing H (1985) Kinder mit posterioren Urethralklappen, Dilatation beider Harnleiter und chronischer Niereninsuffizienz. Urologe [Ausg A] 24: 98–101

Crooks KK (1982) Urethral strictures following transurethral resection of posterior urethral valves. J Urol 127:1153–1154

Egami K, Smith ED (1982) A study of the sequelae of posterior urethral valves. J Urol 127: 84–87

Evins SC, Lorenzo RL (1979) Posterior urethral valves: current concepts in diagnosis and treatment. J Urol 121:76–78

Greenfield SP, Hensle TW, Berdon WE, Geringer AM (1982) Urinary extravasation in the newborn male with posterior urethral valves. J Pediatr Surg 17:751–756

Greenfield SP, Hensle TW, Berdon WE, Wigger HJ (1983) Unilateral vesicoureteral reflux and unilateral nonfunctioning kidney associated with posterior urethral valves – a syndrome? J Urol 130:733–738

Hanna MK, Jeffs RD, Sturgess JM, Barkin M (1977) Urethral structure and ultrastructure. III. The congenitally dilated ureter (megaureter). J Urol 117:24–27

Kurth KH, Alleman ERJ, Schröder FH (1981) Major and minor complications of posterior urethral valves. J Urol 126:517–519

Myers DA, Walker RD (1981) Prevention of urethral strictures in the management of posterior urethral valves. J Urol 126:655–657

Nakayama DK, Harrison MR, de Lorimier AA (1986) Prognosis of posterior urethral valves presenting at birth. J Pediatr Surg 21:43–45

Saalfield JG, Lloyd LK, Evans BB (1976) Management of severe hydroureteronephrosis in infants and young children. J Urol 115:587–590

Vaage S, Stake G, Knutrud O (1974) Obstructive posterior urethral valves. Progr Pediatr Surg 7:125–140

Warshaw BL, Hymes LC, Trulock TS, Woodard JR (1985) Prognostic features in infants with obstructive uropathy due to posterior urethral valves. J Urol 133:240–243

Zaontz MR, Gibbons MD (1984) An antegrade technique for ablation of posterior urethral valves. J Urol 132:982–984

Part II

Corrections of Urinary Transport Disturbances

Microvascular Autotransplantation of Intra-abdominal Testes

P. Frey[1,2] and A. Bianchi[1]

Summary

In the period between 1981 and 1987, 23 microvascular autotransplantations of intra-abdominal testes were performed on 18 patients at the Royal Manchester Children's Hospital. Nineteen testes [82.6%] were successfully revascularised; however, four [17.4%] became partially or totally atrophic. Early surgery is recommended — well before the age of 2 years, prior to the onset of testicular damage, in order to reduce the risk of infertility. Although the early results are very encouraging, only long-term, postpuberty follow-up regarding both fertility and malignancy can determine the value of testicular autotransplantation.

Zusammenfassung

Zwischen 1981 und 1987 wurden am Royal Manchester Children's Hospital 23 mikrochirurgische Autotransplantationen wegen Retentio testis abdominalis an 18 Patienten durchgeführt. 19 Testikel (82.6%) konnten erfolgreich revaskularisiert werden; in 4 (17.4%) Fällen, stellte man eine teilweise oder vollständige Atrophie fest. Es wird empfohlen, den Eingriff vor dem zweiten Lebensjahr durchzuführen, bevor pathologische Veränderungen am Hoden stattfinden können, um dem Risiko der Infertilität vorzubeugen. Obwohl die ersten Ergebnisse sehr vielversprechend sind, müssen die Patienten langfristig beobachtet werden. Nach der Pubertät soll die Fertilität kontrolliert und eine maligne Entwicklung ausgeschlossen werden, erst dann wird man den wirklichen Wert der Autotransplantation der Testikel beurteilen können.

Résumé

Entre 1981 et 1987, 23 autotransplantations microvasculaires de testicules intra-abdominaux ont été pratiquées dans le cas de 18 patients au Royal Manchester Children's Hospital. 19 testicules ont été revascularisés avec succès, soit 82.6%, mais quatre, soit 17.4%, se sont partiellement ou entièrement atrophiés.

[1]Department of Paediatric Surgery, St. Mary's Hospital, and Royal Manchester Children's Hospital, Manchester, United Kingdom
[2]Current address: Kinderchirurgische Klinik, Universitäts-Kinderspital Basel, Römergasse 8, CH-4005 Basel, Switzerland

Progress in Pediatric Surgery, Vol. 23
Ed. by L. Spitz et al.
© Springer-Verlag Berlin Heidelberg 1989

Il est recommandé de pratiquer cette intervention bien avant l'âge de deux ans, c'est-à-dire avant que les testicules aient pu être endommagés avec risque de stérilité. Bien que les résultats soient très encourageants à court terme, il y a lieu de suivre les enfants au-delà de la puberté pour vérifier la fertilité et l'absence d'évolution maligne et juger ainsi de la valeur de l'autotransplantation des testicules.

Introduction

The incidence of cryptorchism is, according to Hadziselimovic (1987), 9.2% in premature babies but 5.8% in full-term boys. Approximately 20% of undescended testes are not clinically palpable (Levitt et al. 1978). They can be either intra-abdominal, intracanalicular, atrophic, dysgenetic or absent; 5%–9% of impalpable testes are indeed either intra-abdominal or absent (Scorer and Farrington 1971). In about 5% of such cases, conventional surgical procedures incorporating extensive retroperitoneal dissection do not succeed in bringing the testis into a scrotal position (Garibyan et al. 1984).

Several operative techniques have been developed to overcome this problem and to avoid orchiectomy. High testicular vessel transection, as described by Fowler and Stephens (1959), is the most commonly practised technique. However, it carries an unacceptable incidence of testicular atrophy of up to 50% (Garibyan et al. 1984). The drastically reduced testicular blood flow, relying only on the artery of the vas deferens, might be sufficient to keep the testis viable but does not guarantee its function (Giuliani et al. 1984).

Similarly, multi-stage orchiopexy as proposed by Corkery (1975) and other authors (Firor 1971; Persky and Albert 1971), in which the testis is brought down into the scrotum in stages, assuming spontaneous elongation of the cord, has shown mixed success. It has been suggested that the additional vessel length achieved by staged orchiopexy reflects inadequate retroperitoneal mobilisation at the primary operation (Redman 1977).

The introduction of microvascular techniques added a new dimension to the operative transposition of intra-abdominal testes. In 1976, MacMahon and co-workers reported successful testicular autotransplantation in mongrel dogs. In the same year, Silber and Kelly (1976) described a successful microvascular autotransplantation of an intra-abdominal testis in a 9-year-old boy. Subsequently, several series of successful autotransplantations of intra-abdominal testes were reported (O'Brien et al. 1983; Upton et al. 1983; Garibyan et al. 1984; Giuliani et al. 1984; Domini et al. 1985; Shiosvilli 1985).

The aims of the treatment of intra-abdominal testes should be:

1. Early transfer of the testis to the scrotum to preserve spermatogonia formation and subsequent spermatogenesis
2. Preservation of hormonal function of the testicular tissue
3. Possible reduction of the risk of malignancy
4. Guarantee of a satisfactory cosmetic result and therefore minimisation of psychological disturbances

Patients

In the period between 1981 and 1987, 23 microvascular orchiopexies were performed on 18 patients. Early results of the first ten cases were reported by Bianchi in 1984. Five patients underwent bilateral procedures. In one child, prune-belly syndrome and in another Noonan's syndrome was diagnosed. In a further patient, the ipsilateral vas and kidney were not present, and in one boy the contralateral testis was congenitally absent. The mean age at primary diagnosis was 1.5 years, (birth–6 years); however, the mean age at referral to the paediatric surgical centre was 4.8 years (1 month–15.25 years). Seven patients had had previous exploratory operations. Eleven patients underwent preoperative laparoscopy, confirming the presence of intra-abdominal testes. Twelve intra-abdominal testes were found on the right side and 11 on the left side. The mean age at operation was 7.4 years, with an age range of 3.25–16 years.

Preoperative Assessment

If a unilateral impalpable testis is diagnosed, it cannot be assumed that it is necessarily absent, as the incidence of monorchia is rare, occurring in one of 5000 males (Burrow and Gough 1970). In case of bilateral impalpable testis, bilateral testicular absence is even more unlikely, as the incidence of anorchia, or true bilateral gonadal agenesis, is extremely low, occurring in one of 20000 males (Burrow and Gough 1970). Therefore, it always becomes necessary to search for an impalpable gonad.

Laparoscopy is by far the most useful investigation, since it definitely confirms the presence of an intra-abdominal testis with a short vascular leash, as well as detecting a blind-ending vas in patients with monorchia, who do not require further treatment. The procedure should be undertaken as an initial investigative event, and further management should be planned on the basis of the laparoscopic findings. The alternative of combining laparoscopy with surgical exploration may lead to unnecessary loss of operative time in the event of monorchia or anorchia. In patients with bilateral non-palpable undescended testis, laparoscopy will be performed only if the presence of testicular tissue has been demonstrated following HCG stimulation.

Ultrasonography, computer tomography and magnetic resonance imaging can be of additional value in detecting the presence and establishing the position of an impalpable testis. Exploratory operations alone should no longer be performed.

Operative Technique

Through a laterally extended groin incision (Fig. 1) the inguinal canal is exposed and the processus vaginalis – gubernaculum identified. The intra-abdominal tes-

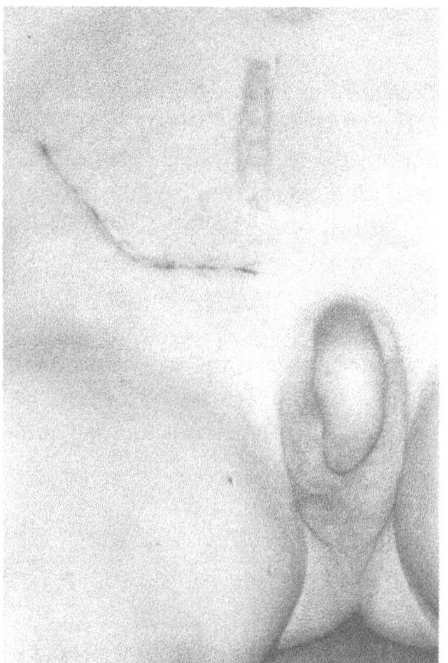 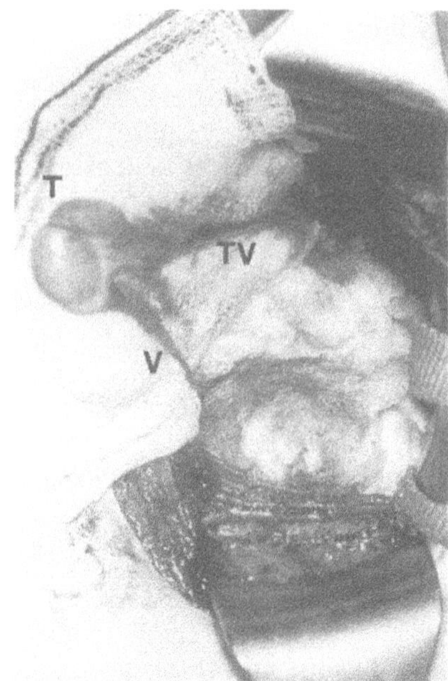

Fig. 1. A laterally extended groin incision gives sufficient exposure to allow a full retroperitoneal dissection of the testicular vessels

Fig. 2. Testis *(T)* after full dissection of testicular vessels *(TV)* and vas *(V)*. Note extremely short vascular leash

tis is brought to an extraperitoneal position and the peritoneum is closed. A full retroperitoneal dissection of the testicular vessels follows, extending approximately to their origin. Figure 2 shows the testis on the fully dissected short vascular leash and the vas deferens. The inferior epigastric vessels are exposed and carefully dissected, using the operating microscope. To gain vascular pedicle length, their division is performed high, beneath the m. rectus abdominis. The testicular vessels are divided high, near their origin. The vessel ends are flushed with heparin solution (10 units to 1 ml normal saline); no systemic antithrombotic agents or hypothermia techniques (Shiosvilli 1985) are used. Under magnification, the testicular artery is anastomosed to the inferior epigastric artery by end-to-end anastomosis using interrupted 10-0 Ethilon sutures on a 3.75-mm, 75-µm needle (W2870). The testicular vein is similarly anastomosed to an inferior epigastric vein (Figs. 3 and 4). The vas is mobilised sufficiently to allow the testis to be placed in a extra dartos pouch without tension. It is occasionally necessary to undertake a full pelvic dissection of the vas to achieve a low scrotal position. A wedge testicular biopsy is performed after revascularisation, thus also allowing a macroscopic assessment of testicular blood flow (Fig. 5). The wound is then closed in layers. Prophylactic antibiotics are administered for 5–7 days postoperatively. Figure 6 schematically illustrates the pre- and postoperative anatomy.

3 4

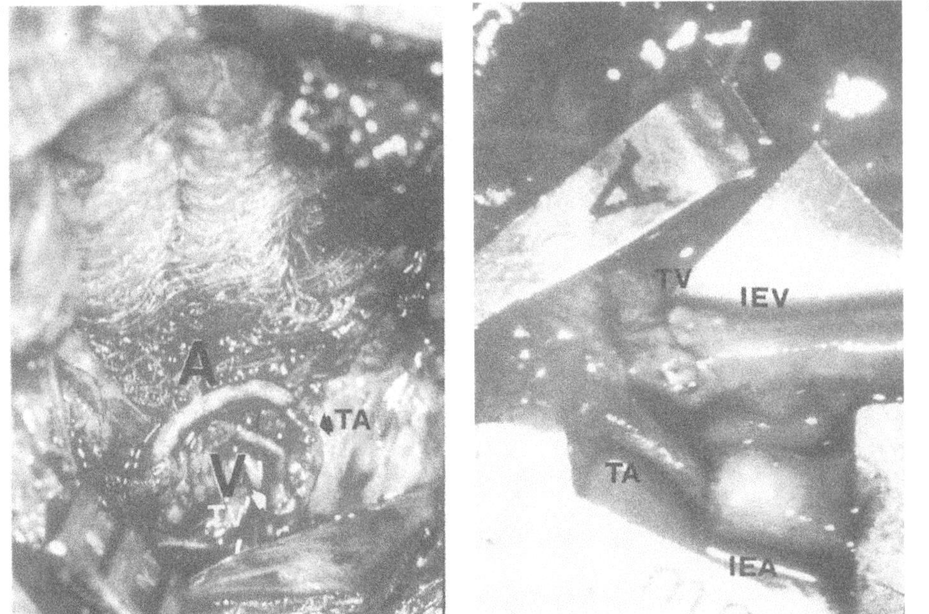

Fig. 3. Testicular artery *(TA)* anastomosed to inferior epigastric artery; testicular vein *(TV)* anastomosed to inferior epigastric vein. Note difference of vascular diameter

Fig. 4. Close up of anastomoses: testicular artery *(TA)* − inferior epigastric artery *(IEA);* testicular vein *(TV)* − inferior epigastric vein *(IEV)*. Note that arteries are still clamped

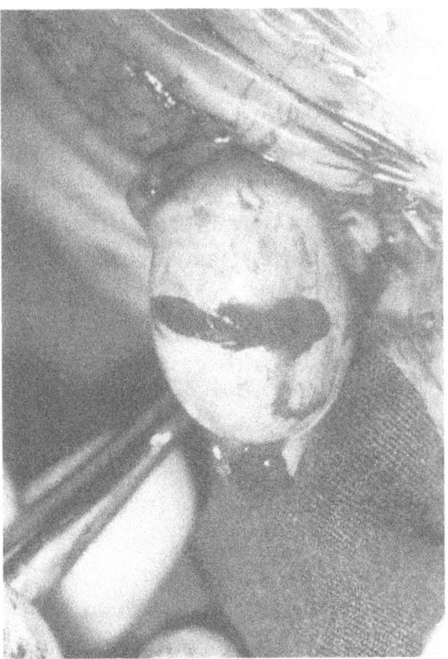

Fig. 5. Macroscopical assessment of blood flow after revascularisation of the testis by incision of the tunica albuginea

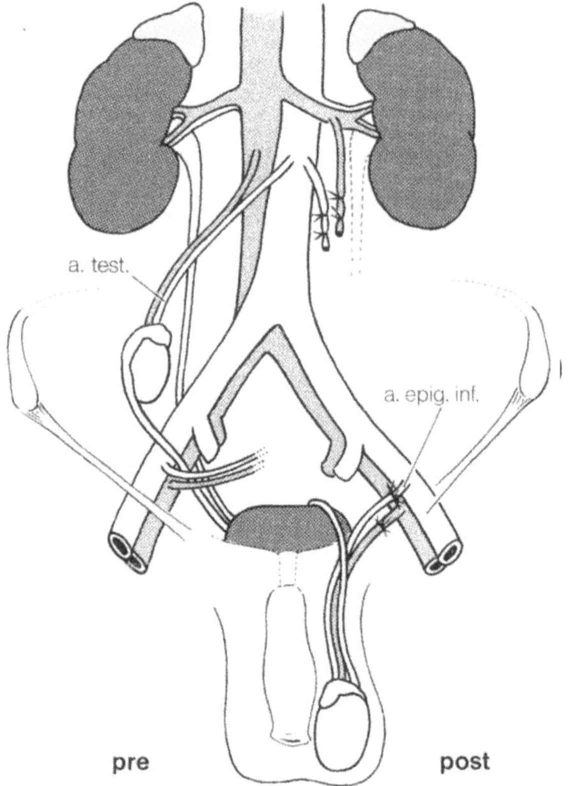

Fig. 6. Anatomy of testes, vas and testicular vessels before *(pre)* and after *(post)* microvascular auto-transplantation

Results

The mean duration of surgery was 4 h. The mean testicular ischaemia time was 1.6 h; however, with experience the operating time was reduced to 2.5–3 h, the ischaemia time to approximately 1 h.

The mean diameter of the testicular artery was 0.6 mm (0.3–0.8 mm) and that of the inferior epigastric artery 1.1 mm (0.8–1.5 mm). The testicular vein showed a mean diameter of 1.3 mm (0.8–3 mm) and the inferior epigastric vein 1.0 mm (0.5–1.5 mm).

Despite the difference in vascular diameter, especially of the arteries, end-to-end anastomosis was possible in all but one case. The immediately postoperative blood flow, macroscopically assessed by bleeding after incision of the tunica albuginea (Fig. 5), was brisk in 21 cases (91%), acceptable in one case (4.5%) and not present in one (4.5%) further case. The average time of hospitalization was 5.9 days, varying from 4 to 10 days.

The follow-up period varied from 1 month to 5.9 years; the mean was 3.3 years. The results of the most recent Doppler flowmetry showed good pulsation over 19 testes (83%) and good pulsation over two testicular arteries (8.5%); however, despite successful microvascular anastomosis, there was failure of testicular development. A further two testes (8.5%) showed reduced or absent pulsation. Following surgery, the size of 17 testes had increased (73.9%), that of two was equal (8.7%), and that of four had decreased (17.4%).

Histological examination of the intraoperative biopsies showed, in all but two cases, the typical picture of underdeveloped testicular tissue with absent spermatagonia. Follow-up histology was performed in only three cases, partly for ethical reasons, but also because its value is questionable prior to puberty. One biopsy, performed 5 months after surgery, showed no histological alteration; a second, 7 months postoperatively, demonstrated a mild improvement in tubular diameter and Sertoli-cell hyperplasia. The biopsy of the third patient, who is in mid puberty, demonstrated improved histology, in that there was an increase in tubular diameter and many healthy-looking Leydig cells were present (not present on the original sections). However, active spermatogenesis was still not seen 1 year postoperatively. The patient and operation data are shown on Table 1, the follow-up results summarised in Table 2.

Discussion

The clinical feasibility of microvascular transfer of intra-abdominal testes is now widely accepted; nevertheless, testicular autotransplantation should be limited to experienced and specialised surgical centres.

In younger children, microvascular anastomosis of vessels with a diameter of at least 0.3 mm no longer represents an insoluble problem. Based both on this and on the histological findings in older children showing severely underdeveloped or damaged gonadal tissue, we are in favour of early operation for intra-abdominal testes to allow testicular development in an optimal scrotal surrounding. This is reinforced by Hadziselimovic's findings (F. Hadziselimovic, personal communication, 1989) that testicular damage resulting in compromised fertility occurs after the second or, in patients with intra-abdominal testis, even after the first year of life. The scrotal positioning of the undescended testis also decreases the incidence of torsion (Bianchi 1984; O'Brien et al. 1983). Unfortunately, there is still a considerable delay in the diagnosis and referral of patients with cryptorchid testes (a mean of 3.3 years in our series).

Despite the higher risk of malignant changes in intra-abdominal testis (Hinman 1979), we do not favour orchiectomy, since the effect of orchiopexy with return of full blood supply before 2 years of age is still unknown. Furthermore, the scrotal testis can be easily examined and testicular changes can be detected early. All patients who have undergone orchiopexy should be taught self-monitoring by regular testicular palpation. Pike and co-workers (1986) state that the age at orchiopexy has no effect on the risk of testicular cancer. However, in their series, only two patients were below the age of 2 years, the majority having had their orchiopexy performed at 10 years or more. Orchiectomy for cancer prophylaxis in patients with bilateral abdominal testis would also deprive the patient of most of

Table 1. Patient and operation data

Patient number	Age at operation (years/months)	Side	Testicular volume (ml)	Operation time (hours)	Ischaemia time (hours)	Histological findings at operation	Hospitalisation (days)	Remarks
1	3³/₁₂	R*	–	4.5	1.5	Not available	5	Absent right vas + kidney
2	6⁵/₁₂	R*	2	5.5	2.25	Poorly formed seminiferous tubules, Sertoli cells, no spermatogonia	7	
	7¹/₁₂	L*	1.5	4	2	Poor, small seminiferous tubules, no lumen, Sertoli cells only, occasional spermatogonia	8	
3	3⁴/₁₂	L*	1	3.25	1.5	220 seminiferous tubules, 15% spermatogonia, no Leydig cells	6	
4	16	L*	5	4	2	Poor, seminiferous tubules, scanty spermatogonia, occasional Leydig cells	7	
5	5¹/₁₂	L*	–	5	–	Not available	7	Failed arterial anastomosis
6	3⁶/₁₂	R*	1.5	5.5	1.25	Early seminiferous tubules, lumen formation, mostly Sertoli cells only, scanty spermatogonia	6	Noonan syndrome
7	13	R*	3	4.5	2	Poor seminiferous tubules, mainly Sertoli cells only, occasional spermatogonia, occasional Leydig cells	7	
8	12⁷/₁₂	R*	–	5.75	2	Poor seminiferous tubules, mostly Sertoli cells, very few spermatogonia, no Leydig cells	10	Prune-belly syndrome
	13½	L*	3	4	1.25	Seminiferous tubules, small lumen, mostly Sertoli cells only, spermatogonia, no Leydig cells	7	

9	3³/₁₂	R*	2	3.5	1.25	Seminiferous tubules, single-layer Sertoli cells, no spermatogonia, no Leydig cells	7	
		L*	2	2.5	1	Small seminiferous tubules, few spermatogonia	5	
10	5⁵/₁₂	L*	1.5	3.5	1.5	Immature seminiferous tubules, no spermatogonia, no Leydig cells	6	
	6⁴/₁₂	R	1.5	3.5	1.5	Hyperplastic seminiferous tubules, single-layer Sertoli cells, no spermatogonia, occasional Leydig cells	5	
11	4⁴/₁₂	R	1.5	4	1.75	Degenerated seminiferous tubules, single-layer Sertoli cells, no viable spermatogonia, no Leydig cells	4	
12	4³/₁₂	R	1.5	5.25	1.75	Immature seminiferous tubules, Sertoli cells only, no spermatogonia, no Leydig cells	4	
13	6½	R	1.5	3.25	1.75	Closely packed with seminiferous tubules, lined by many spermatogonia, no atrophy	5	
14	7⁵/₁₂	L	1.5	3.75	1.25	Immature seminiferous tubules, Sertoni cells only, no spermatogonia	5	Bilateral atrophy
15	12⁷/₁₂	R	5	5.25	1.75	200 seminiferous tubules, lined with Sertoli cells, scanty spermatogonia, no Leydig cells	5	
	13⁴/₁₂	L	7	3	1.75	150 seminiferous tubules, double-layer Sertoli cells, scanty spermatogonia, occasional Leydig cells	5	Only 1 month follow-up
16	9⁹/₁₂	R	2.5	4	2	Not available	5	
17	5⁶/₁₂	L	3	2.5	1	Reduced no. of small seminiferous tubules, Sertoli cells only, no spermatogonia	5	Right testis absent
18	4⁴/₁₂	L	1.5	3.25	1	Seminiferous tubules reduced in diameter and number, no spermatogonia, no Leydig cells	5	

* Early results reported by Bianchi (1984)

Table 2. Follow-up results

Patient number	Follow-up time (years/months)	Location of testis	Condition on palpation	Doppler test		Volume in ml (contralateral)		Follow-up history
				Testis	Spermatic artery			
1	5 9/12	Low scrotal	Atrophic	−	+++	−	(3)	
2	5 5/12	Low scrotal	Normal	+++	+++	5		Increased tubular diameter, hyperplasia, many Sertoli cells, no spermatogonia (improvement)
	4 9/12	Low scrotal	Normal	+++	+++	4		
3	2 9/12	Low scrotal	Normal	+++	+++	2	(3.5)	
4	4	Low scrotal	Normal	+++	+++	5	(3)	
5	4 1/12	Scrotal	Atrophic	−	−	−	(3)	
6	5 5/12	Low scrotal	Normal	+++	+++	4.5	(4)	
7	4 10/12	Low scrotal	Normal	+++	+++	26	(25)	
8	5 11/12	Low scrotal	Normal	+++	+++	20		Reduced no. of seminiferous tubules, Sertoli cells only, occasional spermatogonia, no Leydig cells (no improvement)
	5 5/12	Low scrotal	Normal	+++	+++	20		
9	3 10/12	Low scrotal	Normal	+++	+++	3		
	2 9/12	Low scrotal	Normal	+++	+++	3		
10	3 8/12	Low	Normal	+++	+++	2		
	2 9/12	Scrotal	Normal	+++	+++	2		
11	1 3/12	Low scrotal	Normal	+++	+++	3		
12	5/12	Low scrotal	Normal	+++	+++	3.5	(2)	
13	3/12	Low scrotal	Normal	+++	+++	3.5	(3.5)	
14	3 9/12	Scrotal	Atrophic	−	++	−	(−)	
15	9/12	Low scrotal	Normal	+++	+++	8		Increase in tubular diameter, many Sertoli cells, many Leydig cells, no spermatogenesis (improvement)
	1/12	Low scrotal	Normal	+++	+++	7		
16	2 4/12	Low scrotal	Normal	+++	+++	3	(3)	
17	2 9/12	Low scrotal	Normal	+++	+++	4	(−)	
18	2 9/12	Scrotal	Atrophic	−	++	−	(2.5)	

his endogenous testosterone production and would require permanent hormonal substitution. It could be argued that after successful autotransplantation orchiectomy of the remaining intra-abdominal testis should be performed. However, in our experience, patients with bilateral intra-abdominal testes who have undergone one autotransplantation insist on having the contralateral side operated on.

Despite the possibility of implantation of a testicular prosthesis, the psychological effects of orchiectomy should not be underestimated. A further reason for early restoration of a normal genital appearance, by orchiopexy under any circumstances, is the prevention of an abnormal psychosexual development of the child (Garibyan et al. 1984).

No doubt, only very carefully set up protocols and long-term postpuberty follow-ups, regarding fertility and malignancy as well as psychosexual development, can assess the value of microvascular testicular autotransplantation.

References

Bianchi A (1984) Microvascular orchiopexy for high undescended testes. Br J Urol 56:521–524
Burrow M, Gough MH (1970) Bilateral absence of testes. Lancet 1:366
Corkery JJ (1975) Staged orchiopexy – a new technique. J Pediatr Surg 10:515–518
Domini R, Lima M, Appignani A (1985) Auto-transplantation of the testicle in paediatric utilising microsurgical technique. Z Kinderchir 40:351–354
Firor HV (1971) Two-stage orchiopexy. Arch Surg 102:598–599
Fowler R, Stephens FD (1959) The role of testicular vascular anatomy in the salvage of high undescended testes. Aust NZ J Surg 29:92–106
Garibyan H, Hazebroek FWJ, Schulkes JAR, Molenaar JC, Dabhoiwala NF (1984) Microvascular surgical orchiopexy in the treatment of high-lying undescended testes. Br J Urol 56: 326–329
Giuliani L, Carmignani G, Belgrano E, Puppo P, Trombetta C (1984) Testis auto-transplantation. Prog Reprod Biol Med 10:153–158
Hadziselimovic F (1987) Examination and clinical findings in cryptorchid boys. In: Hadziselimovic F (ed) Cryptorchidism – management and implications. Springer, Berlin Heidelberg New York, pp 93–98
Hinman F (1979) Unilateral abdominal cryptorchidism. J Urol 122:71–75
Levitt SB, Kogan SJ, Engel RH, Weiss RM, Martin DC, Ehrlich RM (1978) The impalpable testis: a rational approach to management. J Urol 120:515–520
MacMahon RA, O'Brien BMcC, Cussen LJ (1976) The use of microsurgery in the treatment of the undescended testis. J Pediatr Surg II:521–526
O'Brien BMcC, Rao VK, MacLeod AM, Morrison WA, MacMahon RA (1983) Microvascular testicular transfer. Plast Reconstr Surg 71:87–90
Persky L, Albert DJ (1971) Staged orchiopexy. Surg Gynecol Obstet 132:43–45
Pike MC, Chilvers C, Peckham MJ (1986) Effect of age at orchidopexy on risk of testicular cancer. Lancet I:1246–1248
Redman JF (1977) The staged orchiopexy: a critical review of the literature. J Urol 117:113–114
Scorer CG, Farrington GH (eds) (1971) Congenital deformities of the testis and epididymis. Appleton-Century-Crofts, New York, p 21
Shiosvilli TI (1985) Bilateral abdominal cryptorchidism in males: auto-transplantation of the testis. Eur Urol 11:386–387
Silber SJ, Kelly J (1976) Successful auto-transplantation of an intra-abdominal testis to the scrotum by microvascular technique. J Urol 115:452–454
Upton J, Schuster SR, Colodny AH, Murray JE (1983) Testicular auto-transplantation in children. Am J Surg 145:514–519

Role of the Kock Pouch in Adolescent Urology

J. Cumming and C. R. J. Woodhouse

Summary

Although cutaneous urinary diversion will continue to have a place in some urological diseases, some patients may benefit from an undiversion. The Kock pouch with a continent reservoir is an alternative where conventional undiversion to the bladder is impossible. Indications, pre-operative preparation, operative technique, results and complications are outlined in detail. In the adolescent patient requiring urinary diversion the Kock pouch should be considered as the last resort. Where reconstruction of the urinary tract is impossible, a continent urinary reservoir by means of the Kock pouch may be indicated.

Zusammenfassung

Obwohl die kutane Urinableitung bei manchen urologischen Erkrankungen noch ihren Stellenwert behält, ist die Rückverlagerung der kutanen Urinableitung bei manchen dieser Patienten indiziert. Hier kann ein sog. Kock-Pouch mit Kontinenz-Reservoir zur Anwendung kommen, wenn die konventionelle Rückverlagerung in die Blase nicht möglich ist. Indikation, präoperative Vorbereitung, Operations-Technik, Ergebnisse und Komplikationen sind im Detail beschrieben. Beim Adoleszenten, der eine Urinableitung benötigt, soll der Kock-Pouch als ultima ratio dienen. Wenn die Rekonstruktion des Harntraktes nicht möglich ist, kann ein Urin-Kontinenz-Reservoir mit der Kock-Pouch-Methode zur Anwendung kommen.

Résumé

Bien que l'urétrostomie cutanée continue à être employée dans le cas de certaines affections urologiques, un replacement de cet abouchement est parfois indiqué pour quelques uns de ces patients. On peut, dans ces cas, envisager une "Kock pouch", donc une poche pour recueillir les urines quand le réabouchement conventionnel dans la vessie n'est pas possible. Les auteurs traitent en détails de l'indication, du traitement préopératoire, de la technique opératoire, des résultats

Institute of Urology, Shaftesbury Hospital, Shaftesbury Avenue, London WC2, UK

Progress in Pediatric Surgery, Vol. 23
Ed. by L. Spitz et al.
© Springer-Verlag Berlin Heidelberg 1989

et des complications éventuelles. Chez les adolescents, la "Kock pouch" ne sera utilisée qu'en dernier ressort. S'il est impossible de reconstituer les voies urinaires, il faudra malgré tout mettre en place une "Kock pouch" pour recueillir les urines.

Introduction

The indications for cutaneous urinary diversion in paediatric urology have changed over the last decade or two, and in the past some patients have had diversions constructed where, with our present knowledge, alternative procedures would have been performed. Although cutaneous urinary diversion will continue to have a place in paediatric urology, it is not without its long-term complications, especially in the upper tract (Neal 1985; Snare et al. 1985; Pernet and Jonas 1985; Orr et al. 1981). In addition, the psychological consequences are important, particularly in the adolescent who is developing and discovering an identity and body image (Jones et al. 1980).

Some patients with cutaneous urinary diversion may be undiverted with the appropriate measures, but there are many in whom a conventional undiversion to the bladder (Gonzales et al. 1986) is impossible. In this group, a continent reservoir can be offered: the Kock pouch is one example.

Method

Construction of the Kock Pouch

The Kock pouch was originally intended to hold intestinal effluent, with a continent outflow valve admitting a large-lumen catheter to allow drainage of the ileal contents (Kock 1971). This pouch has been adapted for use as a urinary reservoir (Kock et al. 1978a, 1982). The principle is to construct a urinary reservoir of ileum. Two "non-return valves" made from intussuscepted ileum maintain continence and prevent ureteric reflux.

Preoperative Preparation

The patient is admitted 3 days before the operation for bowel preparation, full blood count, serum electrolyte estimation and blood crossmatching. The bowel preparation consists of a liquid low-roughage diet and magnesium sulphate (10 ml hourly), continued until clear effluent is achieved. An enema is administered the evening before the operation. Intravenous antibiotic prophylaxis (metronidazole, 500 mg t.i.d. and cefuroxime, 750 mg t.i.d.) is started on induction of anaesthesia and continued for 48 h.

Operative Technique

Skinner et al. (1984) described the technique which we use. Eighty centimetres of distal ileum is mobilised on its mesentery (Fig. 1). The antireflux nipples will be constructed from 17 cm at each end of the ileum. The two middle sections of 22 cm each are sutured together as a "U" and opened along its antimesenteric border (Fig. 2). The antireflux nipples are constructed by creating an intussusception of the middle of the terminal 17 cm so that the inverted nipple will be lying free within the pouch. The important steps in the construction of the antireflux mechanism are:

1. The blood vessels in the mesentery supplying the apex of the intussuscepted ileum are ligated and divided, and a window in the mesentery 5 cm in length is created at this point. This devascularised section is more adherent on its serosal surface and less bulky.
2. The serosal surface of the intussuscepted ileum is superficially incised with the diathermy needle to stimulate adhesion.
3. Once the nipple has been intussuscepted it is held in position by four rows of staples (Autosuture-GIA without a knife; Fig. 3).
4. A T55 stapler is passed into the space between the serosal surfaces of the efferent nipple and the posterior surface of the pouch. This fifth row of staples attaches the nipple to the posterior wall of the pouch to reduce the risk of blowing out the nipple (Fig. 4).
5. We have not used Marlex mesh around the base of the efferent limb in view of the erosive potential experienced by other workers (Boyd et al. 1985). However, we have obtained polyglycolic acid mesh which has been sutured around the base of the nipples to provide a more rigid support for the catheterising channel and, more importantly, to fix the base of the nipple to the wall of the pouch and the abdominal wall (Fig. 5). This reduces the risk of inversion of the nipple and consequent leakage.

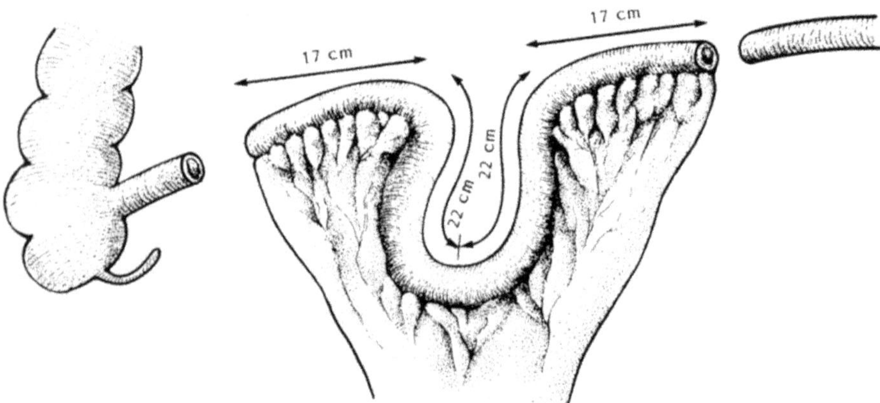

Fig. 1. Eighty centimetres of distal ileum is mobilised on its mesentery. The antireflux nipples will be constructed from 17 cm at each end of the ileum

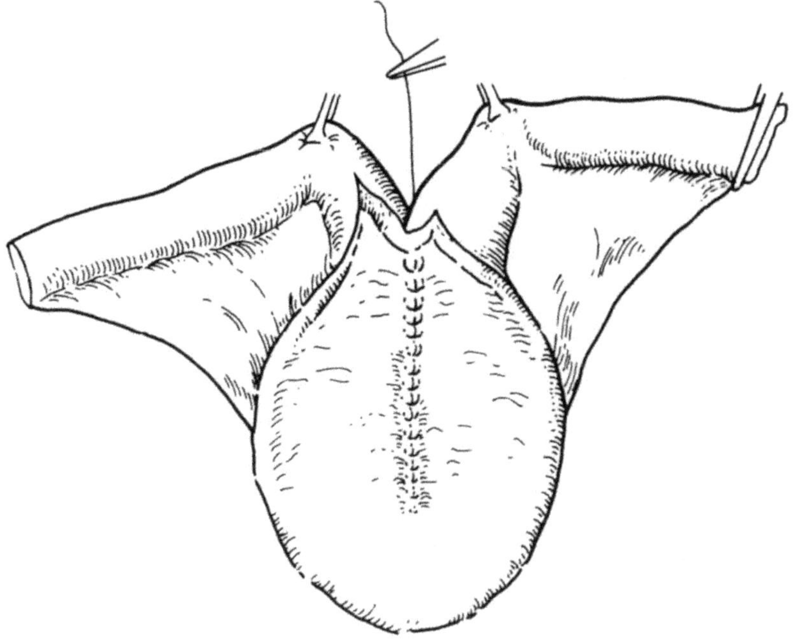

Fig. 2. The two middle sections of 22 cm each are sutured together as a "U" and opened along the antimesenteric border

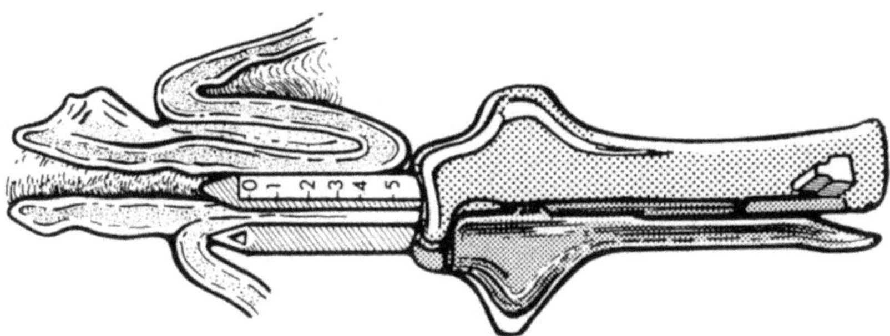

Fig. 3. Once the nipple has been intussuscepted it is held in position by four rows of staples (Autosuture-GIA without a knife)

6. The central limbs, of 22 cm each, are closed to form the storage pouch (Fig. 6).
7. Finally, the ureteric anastomoses (Fig. 7) are splinted with 6F catheters and the pouch is drained continuously with a 28F Foley catheter for 6 weeks to allow the adhesions around the serosal surface of the nipple to develop. The patient then returns to hospital to learn the technique of catheterisation. The pouch gradually expands over the next few weeks to a capacity of 400–1400 ml.

Mucus is produced in intestinal pouches and it drains satisfactorily, assuming a reasonable production of urine is maintained. During the first 10–14 postopera-

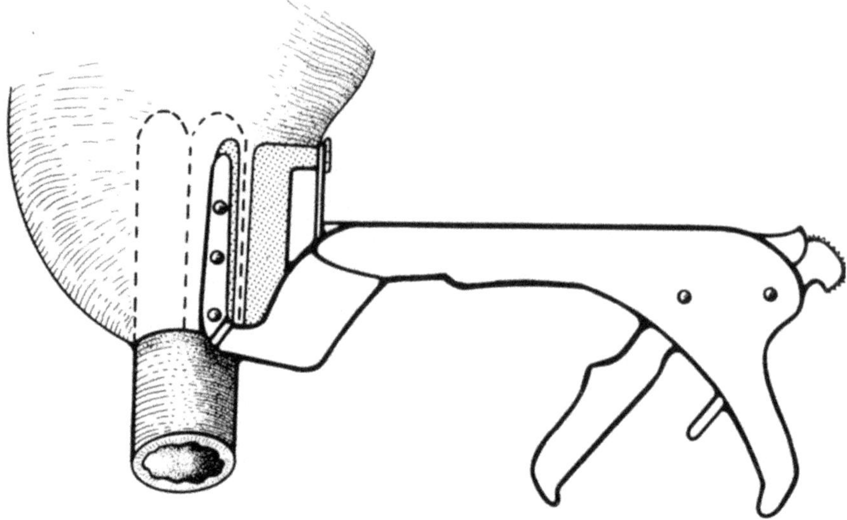

Fig. 4. A T55 stapler is passed into the space between the serosal surfaces of the efferent nipple and the posterior surface of the pouch. This fifth row of staples attaches the nipple to the posterior wall of the pouch to reduce the risk of blowing out the nipple

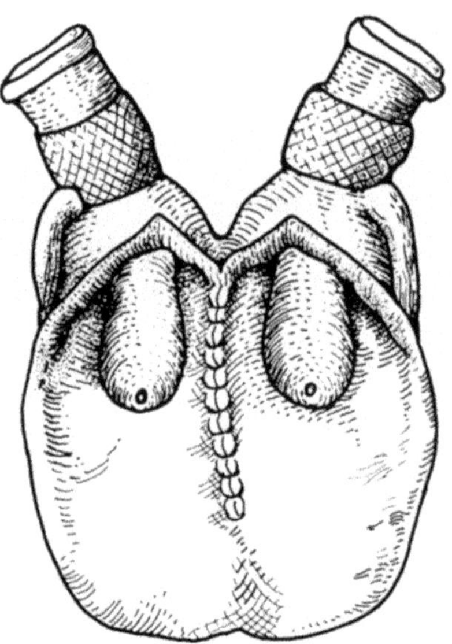

Fig. 5. Polyglycolic acid mesh is sutured around the base of the nipples to provide a more rigid support for the catheterising channel and, more importantly, to fix the base of the nipple to the wall of the pouch and the abdominal wall. This reduces the risk of inversion of the nipple and consequent leakage

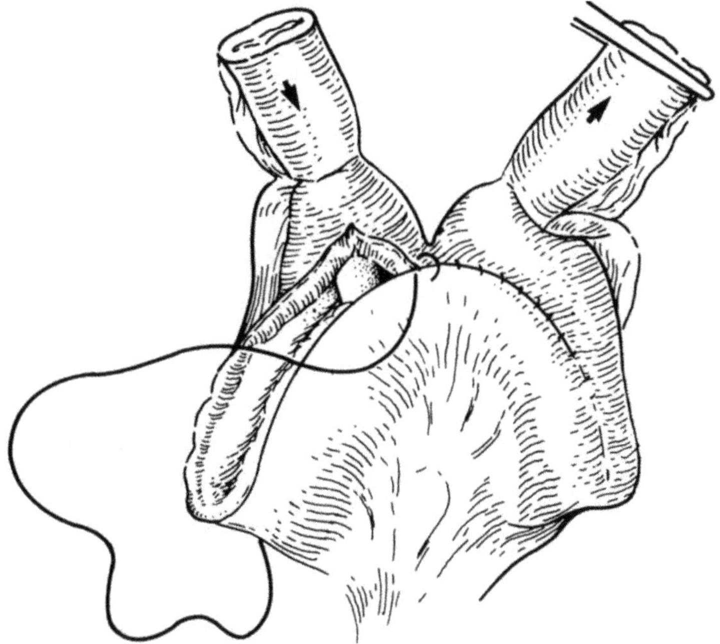

Fig. 6. The central limbs of 22 cm each are closed to form the storage pouch

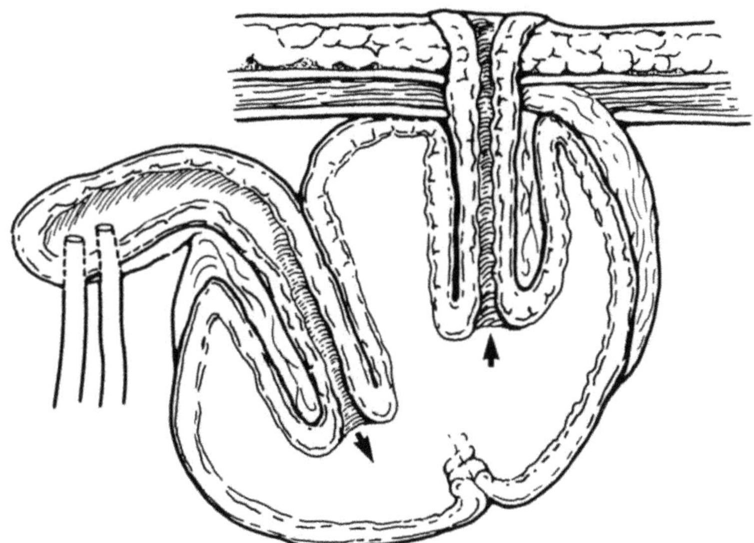

Fig. 7. The efferent limb is anastomosed to the skin and the afferent limb to the ureters. (The ureteric anastomoses are splinted with 6F catheters)

tive days, the Foley catheter is gently irrigated with sterile normal saline twice a day, or more frequently if blockage should occur.

A variation on the Kock pouch has been described by Thuroff and colleagues (1986) called the Mainz pouch. The main difference with the latter is that the terminal ileum and caecum are used. The ureters are implanted into a submucosal tunnel in the caecum. The outflow is controlled by a nipple valve as in the Kock operation. The advantage of this is that the ureteric anastomosis is more satisfactory, but the disadvantage is that haematological complications are likely from vitamin B_{12} malabsorbtion in the long term.

The Place of the Kock Pouch

In the adolescent patient requiring urinary diversion, the Kock pouch should be considered as the last resort. Initially, reconstruction of the urinary tract should be considered. Where this is impossible due to pelvic pathology or absence of the bladder, then a continent urinary reservoir may be considered. We have experience of both the Kock pouch and the Mitrofanoff technique and favour the latter in view of its simpler technique and more reliable results. However, the Mitrofanoff principle relies on using a small calibre tube as the catheterising channel and a tunnelled anastomosis for continence (see Snyder, this volume). There still remain some patients in whom the appendix or fallopian tubes are absent and there is insufficient length of ureter. In these patients who wish to avoid a bag the Kock pouch has its place. Despite the complications that some of our patients have experienced, none has expressed a wish to return to the bag.

Complications

Only one centre in the world has built up a large experience with this procedure (Boyd et al. 1985). The complication rate is high. In a series of 157 patients there were three operative deaths. Early complications, principally fistulae, requiring

Table 1. Details of 12 patients who underwent the Kock pouch operation

No.	Diagnosis
9	Extrophy with urinary diversion
1	Bilateral obstructive megaureter, neuropathic bladder, cystectomy and ileal loop diversion
2	Myelomeningocoele, neuropathic bladder, cystectomy and ileal loop diversion

Table 2. Complications in patients as a result of the Kock pouch operation

No.	Complication
2	Efferent nipple inverting and dilating the nipple and conduit
1	Suture line leak
1	Stenosis of tip of efferent nipple
1	Urinary leak from uretero-ileal anastomosis
1	Anastomotic stenoses

eight reoperations, developed in 24 patients. There were late complications, principally valve failures causing incontinence, in 32 patients. In these 32 patients, 33 reoperations were required. Thus, in expert hands, the major complication rate is 35%. However, the majority of patients were undergoing radical cystectomy for cancer at the same time. In 42 patients, who might be considered the "adolescent" group, the Kock pouch was made for undiversion. It would be reasonable to expect a lower operative complication rate in younger patients, but the valve failure rate is probably the same.

Our experience has been with twelve patients (Table 1). Eight have done well in the short term, with no complications. Four have had major complications requiring ten reoperations but are now well (Cumming et al. 1987; Table 2).

Results

Good results with the Kock pouch require meticulous care with the technique, especially the steps detailed in the construction of the efferent nipple. Our experience and complication rate compares with that of other workers (Boyd et al. 1985; Månsson et al. 1985) and our results have improved with experience. All our patients have been "adolescent" in that their original pathology was congenital, although our oldest patient was 40 years old. None of the continent diversions have been performed for malignancy. In Skinner's department, 60 of the current total of 250 cases have been for undiversion, most in young adults. The complication rate in this group is lower than the average (D. G. Skinner, personal communication).

The benefit of the continent urinary reservoir is mainly the physical and psychological advantage of being rid of the collecting bag. For this reason it is important that the patient is highly motivated.

It is known that, once established, the reservoir is a low-pressure system, with consequent theoretical benefits to the upper tracts (Kock et al. 1978b). However, confirmation of the beneficial long-term effects on renal function must await further follow-up. The reservoir holds 400–1400 ml. Once established, the continence mechanism is reliable, even with stress, in 95% of patients (Boyd et al. 1985). It is emptied by catheter four to five times a day.

A theoretical disadvantage is the loss of 11% of the small bowel, and therefore the loss of some of the absorptive function. However, this remains a theoretical point as none of our patients have suffered from weight loss, diarrhoea or malabsorbtion in the maximum follow-up period fo 3 years. Metabolic and infective complications have not been found in other series or in experimental models (Kock et al. 1985b). The Kock pouch can be made to work, but with difficulty in some patients. There is no doubt that patients with a working pouch much prefer it to an external appliance.

Acknowledgements. We would like to thank Mr. Bartholomew and the Department of Medical Illustration and Photography for their expert assisstance with the illustrations.

References

Boyd SD, Skinner DG, Lieskovsky G (1985) Ongoing experience with the Kock continent ileal reservoir for urinary diversion. World J Urol 3:155–158

Cumming J, Worth PHL, Woodhouse CRJ (1987) The choice of supra-pubic continent catheterisation stoma. Br J Urol 60:227–230

Gonzales R, Sidi AA, Zhang G (1986) Urinary undiversion: indications, technique and results in 50 cases. J Urol 136:13–16

Jones MA, Breckman B, Hendry WF (1980) Life with an ileal conduit: results of questionnaire surveys of patients and urological surgeons. Br J Urol 52:21–25

Kock NG (1971) Ileostomy without external appliances: a survey of 25 patients provided with intra-abdominal intestinal reservoir. Ann Surg 173:545–550

Kock NG, Nilson AE, Norlen L, et al (1978a) Urinary diversion via a continent ileum reservoir: clinical experience. Scand J Urol Nephrol [Suppl] 49:23–31

Kock NG, Nilson AE, Norlen L, et al (1978b) Changes in renal parenchyma and the upper urinary tracts following urinary diversion via a continent urinary diversion. An experimental study in dogs. Scand J Urol Nephrol [Suppl] 49:11–22

Kock NG, Nilson AE, Norlen L, et al (1982) Urinary diversion via a continent ileal reservoir: clinical results in 12 patients. J Urol 128:469–475

Kock NG, Norlen LJ, Philipson BM (1985) Management of complications after construction of a continent ileal reservoir for urinary diversion. World J Urol 3:152–154

Månsson W, Colleen S, Sundin T (1985) Continent caecal reservoir for continent diversion. World J Urol 3:173–178

Neal DE (1985) Complications of ileal conduit diversion in adults with cancer followed up for at least 5 years. Br Med J 290:1695–1697

Orr JD, Shand JEG, Waters DAK, Kirkland IS (1981) Ileal conduit urinary diversion in children. An assessment of the long term results. Br J Urol 53:424–427

Pernet FPPM, Jonas U (1985) Ileal conduit urinary diversion: early and late results of 132 cases in a 25 year period. World J Urol 3:140–144

Skinner DG, Lieskovsky G, Boyd SD (1984) Technique of creation of a continent internal ileal reservoir (Kock pouch) for urinary diversion. Urol Clin North Am 11(4):741–749

Snare J, Walter S, Kristensen JK, Lund F (1985) Ileal conduit urinary diversion – early and late complications. Eur Urol 11:83–86

Thuroff JW, Alken P, Riedmiller H, Engelmann U, Jacobi GH, Hohenfellner R (1986) The Mainz pouch (mixed augmentation ileum and cecum) for bladder augmentation and continent diversion. J Urol 136:17–26

Cloacal Malformations: Embryology, Anatomy and Principles of Management

D. F. M. Thomas

Summary

The cloacal anomaly is characterised by the persistence of a common channel draining the urinary, genital and alimentary tracts via a single orifice. It results from an abnormal compartmentalisation of features that are normal in the primitive female embryo. Abnormal embryology and cloacal anatomy are described in detail. Cloacal abnormalities are usually diagnosed promptly in the neonatal period. Management can be divided into three phases: (1) investigating and defining the anatomy, (2) neonatal intervention with relief of obstruction and (3) definitive surgical reconstruction. Successful management of the child with a cloacal abnormality remains one of the greatest challenges to the pediatric surgeon.

Zusammenfassung

Die Kloaken-Anomalie ist durch die Persistenz eines gemeinsamen Ganges charakterisiert, der den Harn-, Genital- und Verdauungstrakt über eine einzige Öffnung drainiert. Sie resultiert aus einer abnormen Kompartmentierung von Strukturen, die beim jungen weiblichen Embryo zur normalen Entwicklung gehören. Pathologische Embryologie und Anatomie der Kloake werden im Detail beschrieben. Kloakenanomalien werden üblicherweise rasch in der Neugeborenen-Periode diagnostiziert. Das Vorgehen kann in drei Phasen eingeteilt werden: (1) Untersuchung und Klärung der Anatomie, (2) Intervention in der Neonatal-Periode mit Beseitigung von Obstruktionen und (3) endgültige chirurgische Rekonstruktion. Die erfolgreiche Behandlung des Kindes mit einer Kloaken-Anomalie bleibt eine der größten Herausforderungen für den Kinderchirurgen.

Résumé

L'anomalie dite du cloaque est caractérisée par la persistance du canal embryonnaire entoblastique dans lequel continuent à déboucher l'intestin terminal et l'allantoide. Elle est due à un cloisonnement anormal qui constitue une phase normale de l'évolution de l'embryon féminin. Les auteurs traitent en détails des

Department of Paediatric Surgery, St. James's University, Hospital and General Infirmary at Leeds, Belmont Grove, Leeds LS2 9NS, UK

Progress in Pediatric Surgery, Vol. 23
Ed. by L. Spitz et al.
© Springer-Verlag Berlin Heidelberg 1989

aspects embryologiques et de l'anatomie du cloaque. Ce genre d'anomalie est normalement identifié immédiatement chez les nouveaux-nés. Le traitement se fait en règle générale en trois étapes: (1) examen et bilan des données anatomiques, (2) intervention sur le nouveau-né et suppression des obstructions et (3) reconstitution chirurgical définitive. Le succès du traitement d'un enfant présentant une anomalie du cloaque reste un défit majeur pour le chirurgien pédiatrique et il ne manquera pas de le relever.

Introduction

The cloacal anomaly is characterised by the persistence of a common channel draining the urinary, genital and alimentary tracts via a single perineal orifice. To understand the complex anatomy of this lesion it is helpful to consider its embryological derivation.

Normal Embryology

The presence of a common channel or cloaca is a normal feature of the primitive female embryo, but by 3½ weeks a process of compartmentalisation has already begun. The urorectal septum descends towards the perineum to separate the cloaca into urogenital sinus anteriorly and rectum posteriorly − a process which is complete by the 7th week (Fig. 1). By the 8th week, the paired Müllerian (paramesonephric) ducts have made their appearance and have begun to descend caudally and medially in the direction of the urogenital sinus. (Fig. 2). The Müllerian ducts will ultimately form the Fallopian tubes, uterus and major part of the vagina. At 10 weeks the Müllerian ducts fuse and merge with the urogenital sinus in the midline to form the Müllerian tubercle which, in turn, generates the cells of the vaginal plate (Fig. 3). From the 10th to the 20th week the vaginal plate proliferates, extends caudally and then canalises to form the vagina (Fig. 4). This pro-

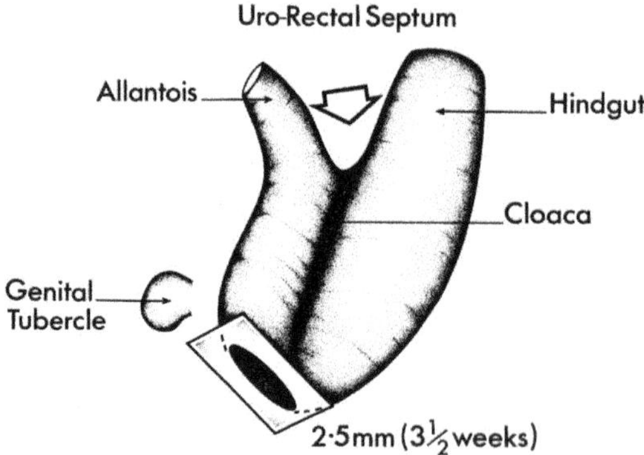

Fig. 1. Normal descent of urorectal septum

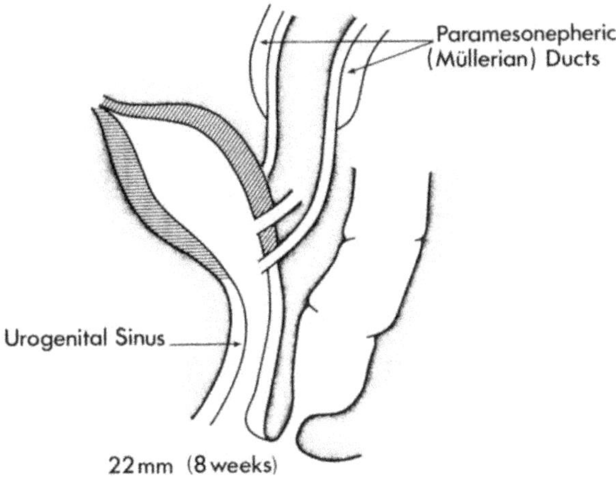

Fig. 2. Appearance of paired Müllerian (paramesonephric) ducts

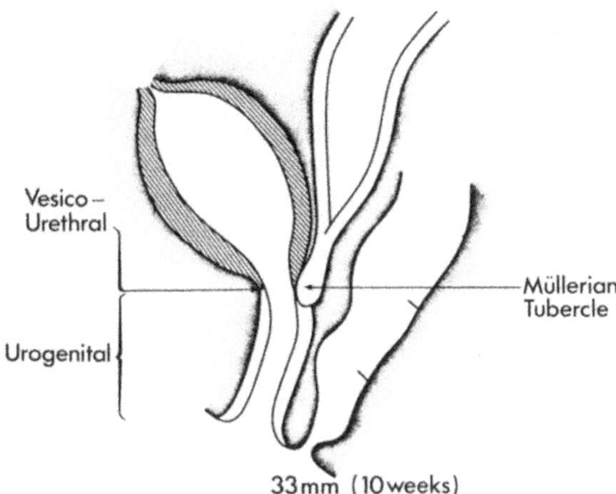

Fig. 3. Formation of Müllerian tubercle

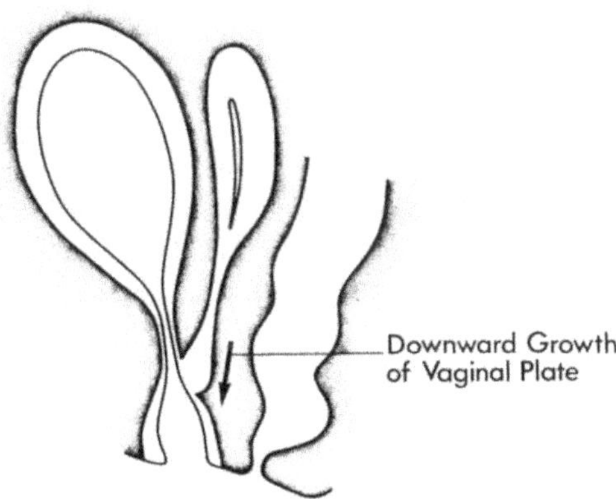

Fig. 4. Proliferation and canalisation of vaginal plate

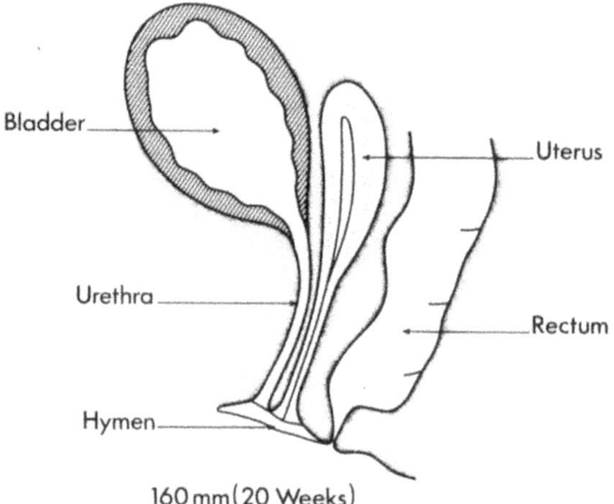

Fig. 5. Definitive female anatomy established

cess is accompanied by change in the relative proportions of the urogenital sinus above and below the Müllerian tubercle. The section of urogenital sinus above the Müllerian tubercle increases in relative length to form the definitive urethra, whilst below the Müllerian tubercle the urogenital sinus undergoes relative regression and is finally represented only by the introitus, the hymen and possibly by a short length of distal vagina. The definitive female genital anatomy is established by 20 weeks (Fig. 5).

Abnormal Embryology: Cloacal Anatomy

It is not difficult to envisage that the cloacal abnormality might arise from an early failure of the urorectal septum to descend and compartmentalise the primitive common channels. A persisting high fistulous communication between the rectum and urogenital sinus would form a barrier to the migrating Müllerian ducts and would prevent them from fusing normally in the midline (Fig. 6). This mechanism is consistent with the observed association between vaginal and uterine duplication and cloacal abnormalities. The disordered embryology of cloacal malformations is considered in detail by Johnson et al. (1972).

In a typical term infant with a cloaca, the visible anomaly consists of the opening of the urogenital sinus at the base of a rudimentary phallus in an otherwise featureless perineum. The internal anatomy of a high-confluence cloaca (Fig. 7) comprises a supralevator fistula connecting the blind-ending rectum to the upper portion of the urogenital sinus. The vagina (which is frequently septate) forms the third element of the confluence. Impaired drainage of the high vagina often results in the accumulation of secretions or retrograde filling with urine causing massive distension (hydrocolpos). Hydronephrosis and hydroureter is another relatively common finding due either to gross vesico-ureteric reflux or to ureteric

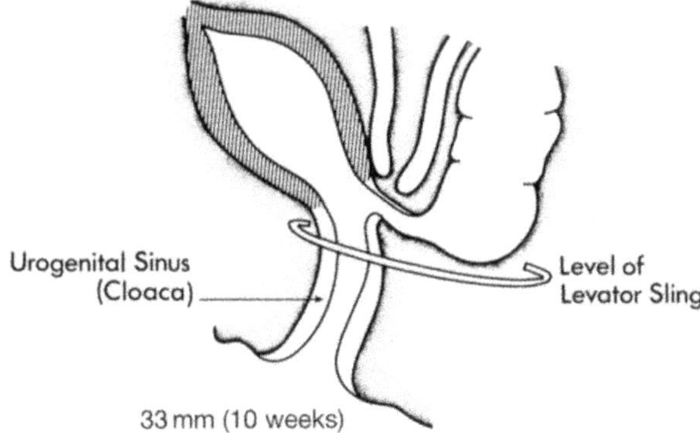

Fig. 6. Failed descent of uro-rectal septum — sino-rectal fistula preventing fusion of the Müllerian ducts

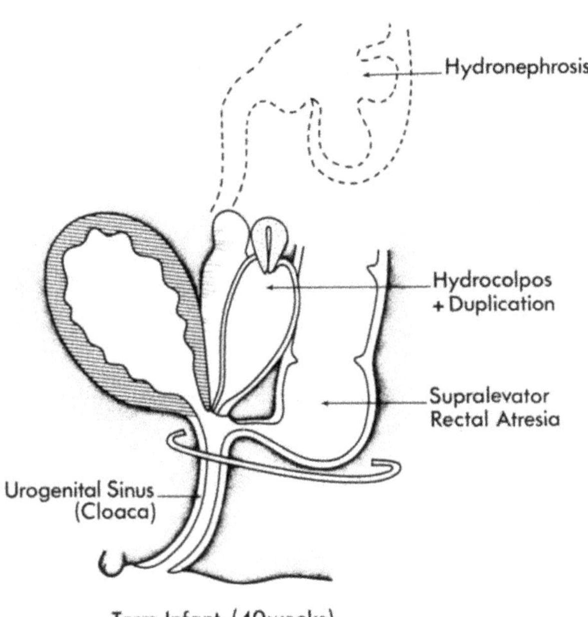

Fig. 7. Internal anatomy of high confluence cloacal anomaly

obstruction from extrinsic compression (by the hydrocolpos) or intrinsic stenosis associated with ectopic drainage.

The high-confluence cloacal anatomy represents the most severe manifestation of incomplete descent of the urorectal septum (Fig. 8). In a less severe form the common channel may be relatively short and the confluence of the urinary, genital and alimentary tracts may lie below the level of the levator mechanisms. In some infants the abnormality is confined to the presence of a urogenital sinus associated with an anterior ectopic anus. It is not clear whether a urogenital sinus in the presence of a normally sited anus is part of the spectrum of urorectal septum defects or whether it represents a different embryological mechanism.

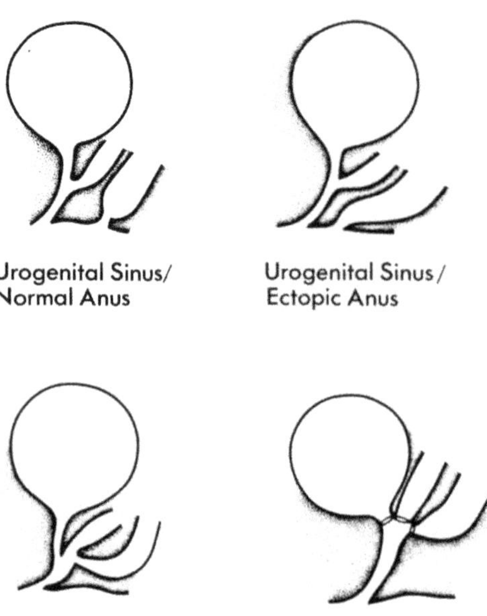

Urogenital Sinus/
Normal Anus

Urogenital Sinus/
Ectopic Anus

Low (Infralevator)
Confluence

High (Supralevator)
Confluence

Fig. 8. Spectrum of cloacal anomalies

Clinical Presentation

Cloacal abnormalities are usually diagnosed promptly in the neonatal period following the discovery of a single perineal orifice. The absence of a hymen is an important diagnostic feature. Hydrometrocolpos may be evident as a visible or palpable lower abdominal mass arising out of the pelvis.

Surgical Management

Surgical management can be conveniently divided into three broad phases:

Investigation: Defining the Anatomy. The aim of investigation is to establish the level at which the urinary, genital and alimentary tracts fuse and to determine their relationship to the levator ani and the urinary sphincter mechanism. In the neonatal period this information is required to allow the surgeon to identify and relieve any obstruction that is present. At a later stage more detailed investigation will be necessary to plan definitive reconstructive surgery. The maximum amount of anatomical information will be obtained by a combination of ultrasound imaging, contrast radiology with screening (fluoroscopy) and direct visualisation by endoscopy. However, despite the use of a full range of modern imaging tech-

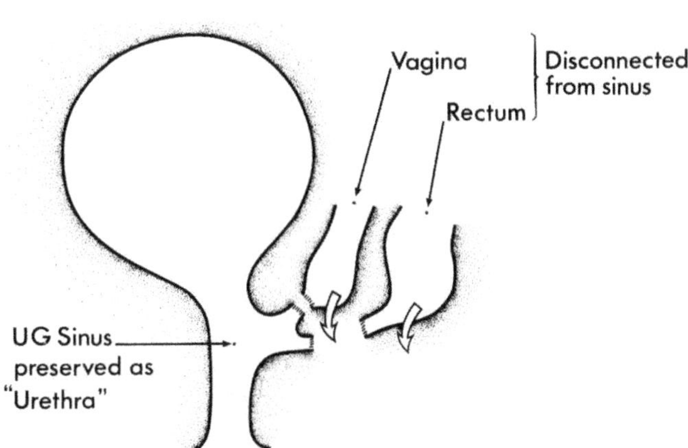

Fig. 9. Basics of reconstructive surgery: isolating rectum and vagina. *UG,* urogenital

niques the true anatomy of some of the more complex lesions may only become apparent at the time of operation.

Neonatal Intervention: Relief of Obstruction. Almost every neonate with a cloacal anomaly will require a defunctioning colostomy in the first few days of life. The need to relieve obstruction in the urinary and genital tracts is sometimes less obvious. Hendren (1982) has stressed the role of unrelieved urinary tract obstruction as a potent cause of death and morbidity in this condition. The urinary tract obstruction is often secondary to the hydrocolops. Therapeutic options include: (a) intermittent catheterisation of the urogenital sinus, (b) exteriorisation of the vagina in the neonatal period, e.g. the vaginal pull-through technique described by Raffensperger and Ramenofsky (Ramenofsky 1980) and (c) suprapubic cystostomy or nephrostomy. Although total correction of the defect in the neonatal period has been described, it is the general view that reconstructive surgery is best deferred until the child is around 6–12 months of age. Hendren (1982), with his extensive personal experience of the management of this condition, cautions against definitive surgery in the neonatal period, stating that "I have not seen a case where that seemed to be the best course." Therefore, once adequate drainage of the obstructed tracts has been established, most infants may leave hospital pending their readmission for definitive surgery at a later date.

Reconstruction Surgery. The precise requirements of any reconstructive procedure will depend upon the particular anatomy of the affected infant. Nevertheless, most operations include the following basic components (Figs. 9, 10; Hendren 1982; Ramenofsky 1980; Henchen 1980; Hecker 1985):

1. The vagina is separated from the urogenital sinus. It will then be necessary to ensure that the vagina drains adequately into the perineum. This can be done

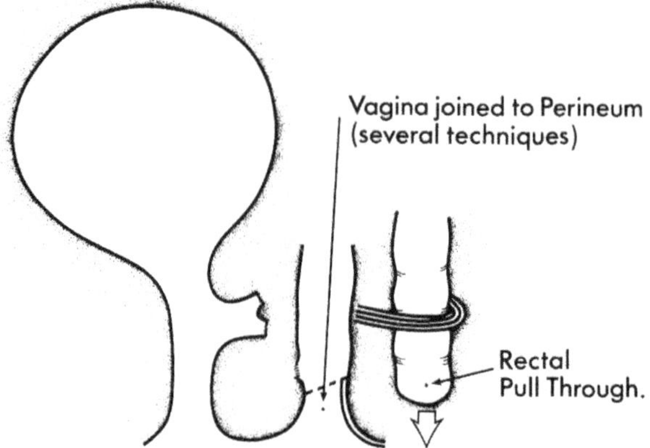

Fig. 10. Basics of reconstructive surgery: vaginal reconstruction and rectal pull-through

by mobilising the vagina and taking it down to the perineum, e.g. by the vaginal pull-through technique (Ramenofsky 1980) or by taking a generous posteriorly based perineal flap up towards the high vagina. Alternatively, a combination of both techniques may be required. Vaginal substitution, e.g. with a segment of small or large intestine, may be necessary if the vagina is too high or too small to be joined adequately to the perineum by the methods described above. Vaginal substitution may also be necessary as a salvage procedure where previous vaginal surgery has failed.

2. The fistula joining the atretic rectum to the urogenital sinus is divided. Some form of abdomino-perineal pull-through procedure (high confluence cloaca) or limited mobilisation and perineal pull-through (for a low confluence anomaly) will then be required.

3. The urogenital sinus is preserved to function as a urethra.

Assessing the Results of Surgery

The relative rarity of cloacal anomalies is such that only a handful of paediatric surgeons are likely to acquire meaningful personal series of these cases during their professional careers. Furthermore, the range of anatomical variants that may be encountered and the number of different surgical options makes it difficult, if not impossible, to quantify the outcome of surgical intervention or to compare the relative success rates of different techniques. Hendren (1982) reviewed 35 cases treated by him and concluded that "most can be reconstructed to achieve satisfactory function." Failed or unsuccessful reconstructive surgery may result in life-long faecal and urinary incontinence (or cutaneous diversions) and a denial of normal sexual and reproductive activity. Thus, the successful management of the child with a cloacal abnormality remains one of the greatest challenges to the paediatric surgeon.

References

Hecker WC (1985) Surgical correction of intersexual genitalia and female genital malformation. Springer, Berlin Heidelberg New York, pp 96–107

Hendren WH (1980) Urogenital sinus and anorectal malformation: experience with 22 cases. J Pediatr Surg 15:628–641

Hendren WH (1982) Further experience in reconstructive surgery for cloacal anomalies. J Pediatr Surg 17(6):695–715

Johnson RJ, Packen M, Derrick W, Bill AH (1972) The embryology of high anorectal and associated genito-urinary anomalies in the female. Surg Gynecol Obstet 135:759–763

Ramenofsky ML (1980) Vaginal lesions. In: Holder TM, Ashcraft KW (eds) Paediatric surgery. Saunders, Philadelphia, pp 902–903

Genitoplasty for Congenital Adrenal Hyperplasia: Anatomy and Technical Review

R. H. Whitaker

Summary

There is variable virilisation in female pseudohermaphrodites with congenital adrenal hyperplasia, but they always have normal ovaries, uterus and upper part of the vagina. The various anatomical stages of virilisation are outlined and a historical review is given. For psychological and practical reasons it is generally accepted that the operation should be performed when the patient is between 6 and 18 months of age. The aim is to reduce the size of the clitoris and to expose the vagina so that it opens onto the perineum. Operative procedures are described. The child is reviewed at intervals to determine the size and shape of the vagina and clitoris. Adjustments can be made around the time of puberty but are rarely necessary.

Zusammenfassung

Weibliche Pseudohermaphroditen mit adrenogenitalem Syndrome zeigen eine Virilisation verschiedenen Ausmaßes, jedoch besitzen sie immer normale Ovarien, Uterus und obere Vagina. Die Anatomie der einzelnen Virilisationsgrade wird dargelegt und ein historischer Überblick gegeben. Aus psychologischen und praktischen Gründen soll die Operation anerkanntermaßen zwischen dem 6. und 18. Lebensmonat durchgeführt werden. Das Ziel der Operation ist eine Reduktion der Clitorisgröße und eine Darstellung der Vagina, so daß diese in den Damm mündet. Die Operationstechniken werden beschrieben. Das Kind wird regelmäßig nachuntersucht, um die Größe und Form von Vagina und Clitoris zu verfolgen. Korrekturen können um die Pubertätszeit vorgenommen werden, sind aber selten erforderlich.

Résumé

Le pseudohermaphrodisme féminin avec hyperplasie surrénale congénitale entraîne une virilisation plus ou moins prononcée mais les ovaires, l'utérus et la partie supérieure du vagin sont normaux. Les auteurs décrivent les caractéristiques anatomiques des différents degrés de virilisation et donnet un aperçu de l'évolu-

Department of Urology, Addenbrooke's Hospital, Cambridge, CB2 2QQ, UK

Progress in Pediatric Surgery, Vol. 23
Ed. by L. Spitz et al.
© Springer-Verlag Berlin Heidelberg 1989

tion. Pour des raisons pratiques autant que psychologiques, cette intervention est généralement pratiquée entre 6 et 18 mois. Elle visera à réduire la taille du clitoris et à modifier le vagin de façon à ce qu'il débouche dans le périnée. Les techniques opératoires sont décrites. On suivra l'enfant et on pratiquera des examens réguliers pour vérifier taille et forme du vagin et du clitoris. Il est possible, le cas échéant, de procéder à des corrections à la puberté mais cela s'avère rarement nécessaire.

Introduction

There is variable virilisation in female pseudohermaphrodites with congenital adrenal hyperplasia, but the ovaries, uterus and upper part of the vagina are always normal. Minimal virilisation comprises a slightly enlarged clitoris with fused labia, whereas in severe virilisation the external genitalia may resemble those of a normal cryptorchid boy. A description of the biochemical defects and their initial management are outside the scope of this surgical review.

Anatomy

Figure 1a shows the anatomy in the least virilised female child, where the urogenital sinus is short and the urethra opens in an almost normal position. The

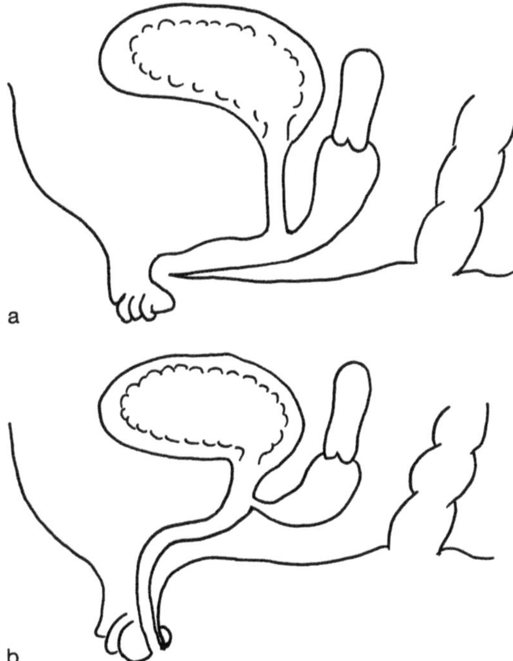

Fig. 1.a Low confluence of vagina and urethra in lesser degrees of virilisation. b High upper vagina connecting through into the posterior urethra. Severe form of virilisation

vagina is easily accessible surgically. In some of these children with minimal clitoral hypertrophy, little more is needed than a simple cutback. In Fig. 1b the vagina enters the posterior urethra high up and this represents the severest form of virilisation, in which the clitoris is usually large and the urogenital sinus may extend to the tip of the phallus and resemble a normal urethra. Fortunately, this latter type is rare, as the surgery is difficult and the results are less satisfactory.

Historical Review

Jones and Scott (1971) stated that Neugebauer reported incising the urogenital sinus in 1908 but no reference was given. Young (1937) gave an accurate description of the condition and a procedure to deal with it. He incised the sinus vertically and removed the clitoris completely, leaving a piece of ventral mucosa in its place. Although Money et al. (1955) reported that the clitoris was not necessary for orgasm, others believed that it should be kept and simply be recessed to a neater shape and size. Thus, Lattimer (1961) described an operation for the relocation and recession of the clitoris as an alternative to amputation. A slightly different operation was later reported by Randolph and Hung (1970).

Approximation of the cut edge of the perineum to the vaginal wall was a problem in these early operations, and Fortunoff et al. (1964) suggested a U- or V-shaped flap, posteriorly based, to be inserted into the posterior aspect of the vagina after its exposure. A further advance was proposed by Goodwin (1969) who suggested that the glans should be preserved, but the corpora cavernosa beneath is removed. However, Williams had already stated in his textbook (Newns and Williams 1968) that this type of clitoral reduction, with a vaginoplasty using the U-shaped flap, was his current technique.

Hendren and Crawford (1969) described in detail the problem of the high vagina that enters the posterior urethra. They advocated a pull-through operation for this rare form of virilisation to facilitate access to the vagina and to avoid the risk of damaging the urinary sphincters.

In 1971, despite these advances, Jones and Scott (1971) were still advocating a vertical perineal incision and a complete clitorectomy. However, they accepted that a U-shaped incision was helpful in the difficult cases. Marberger (1972), as quoted by Allen (1976), was the first to use the prepuce to reconstruct the labia. He resected the clitoris, but was still using a vertical incision to expose the vagina. Spence and Allen (1973) gave a clear description of their own technique but they were still not using the prepuce for the labia.

The technique that many use today, described below, has evolved from the experience of several surgeons. Whitaker (1981) and Grant and Johnston (1982) discussed it without giving any historical details. Recently, attempts have been made to simplify the clitoral reduction and Glassberg and Laungani (1981) suggested that the phallus can be lessened in size by a series of wedge excisions. A more ingenious approach was put forward by Kogan et al. (1983) who remove the erectile tissue from within the corpora cavernosa, but otherwise leave the tunica intact.

Surgical Management

For psychological and practical reasons it is now accepted that the operation should be performed on patients between 6 and 18 months of age, but there is some doubt as to whether the child with a high vagina should be operated so young. Extra steroids, and perhaps salt, are needed throughout the operative and postoperative period.

The aim is to reduce the size of the clitoris and to expose the vagina so that it opens onto the perineum. To achieve the best access, the child should be placed in the lithotomy position. In children with minimal virilisation a cutback may be all that is necessary. This will separate the labia and expose the urethra. The clitoris may, or may not, need reducing.

Vaginoplasty

For more severe forms of virilisation the approach is via a posteriorly based U- or V-shaped flap (Fig. 2, 3). The sinus is then incised until first the urethra is exposed and then, further back, the vagina is encountered (Fig. 3, 4). It is most important to extend the incision in the posterior wall of the vagina until its widest part is reached, as this lessens the risk of later stenosis (Fig. 4). The tip of the skin flap

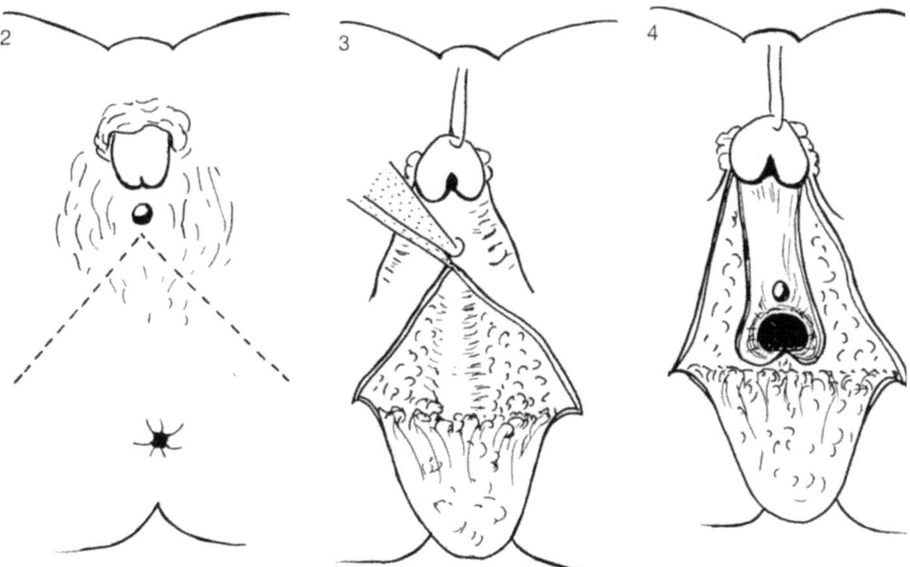

Fig. 2. V-shaped incision with posterior base

Fig. 3. Incision of the sinus

Fig. 4. Exposure of the vagina with incision up to its widest aspect

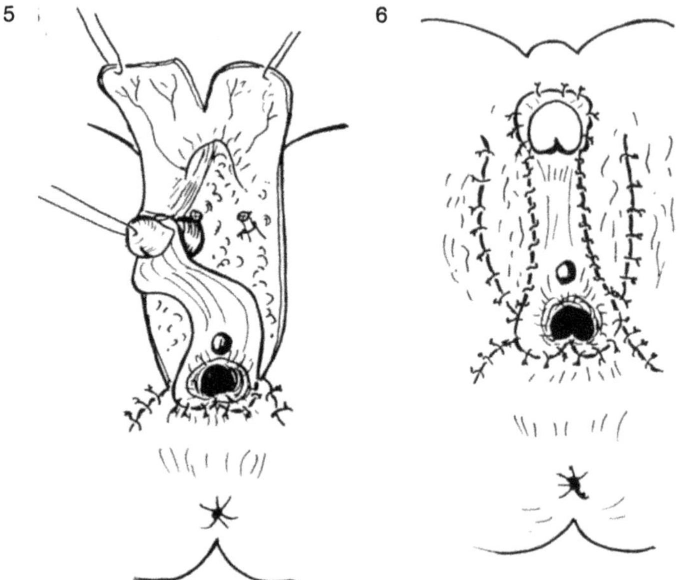

Fig. 5. Isolation of the glans with its dorsal neurovascular bundle and ventral mucosal strip. The preputial skin has been incised in the midline

Fig. 6. The preputial skin has been sutured alongside the mucosal strip to give labia minora

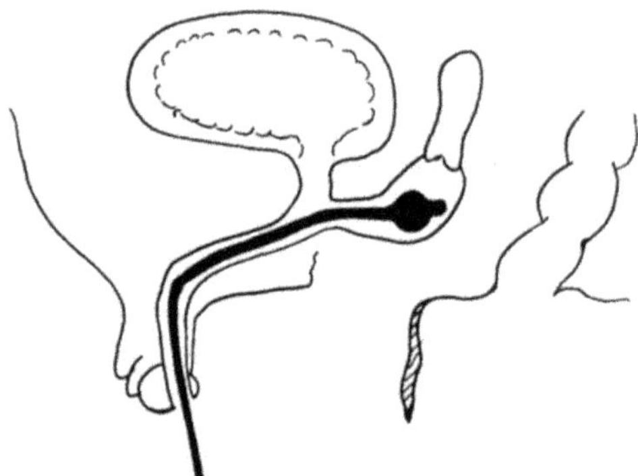

Fig. 7. Fogarty catheter in the high vagina to facilitate later dissection

is then sutured into the posterior incision in the vagina with Dexon or chromic catgut (Fig. 5, 6).

In the child with a high vagina opening into the posterior urethra, the connection must be identified endoscopically before surgery is commenced. A small balloon catheter (Fogarty) can be inserted into the vagina and inflated, giving a good guide for the identification of the vagina later in the procedure (Fig. 7). In this type of high lesion, the sinus is then incised until the normal position of the

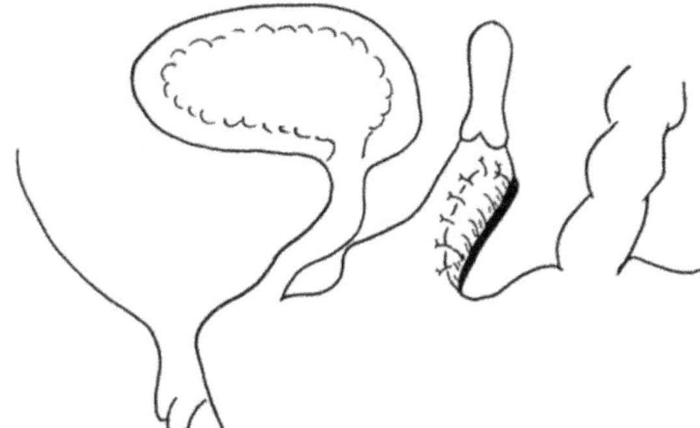

Fig. 8. The urethra is formed by the posterior part of the sinus when there is a high vagina. The skin flap has been laid into the posterior part of the opened vagina

urethra is reached. The skin edges are then sewn to the edges of the sinus to make an external urethral meatus, and all the sinus above this point remains as the proximal urethra. The dissection thereafter is all behind this area and the balloon is identified high up in front of the rectum. An incision is then made in the most anterior part of the vagina so that there is as much length as possible to suture to the posterior skin flap. The bulky skin flap is spread around to cover as much of the denuded area as possible within the vagina (Fig. 8). The lower, anterior part of the vagina can be covered, at least to some extent, by the posterior limits of the preputial skin.

Clitoral Reduction

The phallus is then reduced. The strip of mucosa anterior to the urethra is preserved together with the glans and the dorsal neurovascular bundle. An incision is made around the glans, leaving a generous width of mucosa. This exposes the corpora. The bundle is dissected off the dorsal aspect, together with a strip of tunica, to avoid damaging it. Similarly, the ventral mucosal strip is dissected away from the corpora. The corpora are then traced and dissected to their origins and ligated. A small stub of corpora is left attached to the glans for ease of suturing it to the under-surface of the pubic arch.

The preputial hood is divided at its midline and laid backwards to form the labia minora (Fig. 6). In the child with a high vagina, the distal tips of the preputial skin can be used to line the anterior aspect of the vagina. It is fortunate that in such children there is usually plenty of phallic skin for this purpose. A running suture must be used for the anastomosis of the mucosa to the preputial skin as the spongy tissue can, on occasions, bleed excessively.

A drain is necessary in each side of the wound for 24 h and a urethral catheter for about 3 days. The vagina is packed with vaseline gauze for 48 h and, as soon as it is removed, vaginal dilatation is commenced with a small plastic dilator until the whole wound is fully healed, which takes approximately 1 month.

Follow-up

The child is reviewed at intervals and, around the time of puberty, the area is inspected under anaesthesia. The size and shape of the vagina and clitoris are determined. Adjustments can be made at this stage, but are rarely necessary. A clitoris that seemed too large at the time of the operation often looks more satisfactory later.

References

Allen TD (1976) Reconstruction of the female with ambiguous genitalia. In: Kelalis PP, King LR (eds) Clinical pediatric urology. Saunders, Philadelphia, pp 1023–1028

Fortunoff S, Lattimer JK, Edson M (1964) Vaginoplasty technique for female hermaphrodites. Surg Gynecol Obstet 118:545–548

Glassberg KI, Laungani G (1981) Reduction clitoroplasty. Urology 17:604–605

Goodwin WE (1969) Anomalies of the genitourinary tract. In: de la Camp HB, Linder F, Trede M (eds) American College of Surgeons and Deutsche Gesellschaft für Chirurgie (Joint meeting, Munich, 1968). Springer, Berlin Heidelberg New York, p 256

Grant DB, Johnston JH (1982) Congenital adrenal hyperplasia and female pseudohermaphroditism. In: Williams DI, Johnston JH (eds) Paediatric urology, 2nd edn. Butterworth, London, pp 525–536

Hendren WH, Crawford JD (1969) Adrenogenital syndrome: the anatomy of the anomaly and its repair; some new concepts. J Pediatr Surg 4:49–58

Jones HW, Scott WW (1971) Construction of the feminine external genitalia. In: Jones HW, Scott WW (eds) Hermaphroditism, genital anomalies and related endocrine disorders, 2nd edn. Williams and Wilkins, Baltimore, pp 335–348

Kogan SJ, Smey P, Levitt SB (1983) Subtunical total reduction clitoroplasty: a safe modification of existing techniques. J Urol 130:746–748

Lattimer JK (1961) Relocation and recession of the enlarged clitoris with preservation of the glans: an alternative to amputation. J Urol 86:113–116

Money J, Hampson JG, Hampson JL (1955) Hermaphroditism: recommendations concerning assignment of sex, change of sex and psychologic management. Bull Johns Hopkins Hosp 97:284–300

Newns GH, Williams DI (1968) Abnormalities of sexual development. In: Williams DI (ed) Paediatric urology. Butterworths, London, pp 486–520

Randolph JG, Hung W (1970) Reduction clitoroplasty in females with hypertrophied clitoris. J Pediatr Surg 5:224–231

Spence HM, Allen TD (1973) Genital reconstruction in the female with the adrenogenital syndrome. Br J Urol 45:126–130

Whitaker RH (1981) Reconstruction of the genitalia in the adrenogenital syndrome: In: Westenfelder M, Whitaker RH (eds) Malformations of the external genitalia. Monographs in paediatrics. Karger, Basel, pp 86–88

Young HH (1937) Genital abnormalities, hermaphroditism and related adrenal diseases. Williams and Wilkins, Baltimore

Surgical Correction
of Virilised Female External Genitalia

J. Engert

Summary

Recent investigations and reports on late results indicate that vaginal orgasm is more the exception than the rule, so that, for a woman, preservation of clitoral sensitivity is essential to a satisfying sexual life. All techniques involving total clitoridectomy, plastic imitations, or displacement of the clitoris under the symphysis must therefore be discarded. Even if plication or trapping of an enlarged clitoral shaft under the mons veneris can be regarded as sensitivity-maintaining procedures, they nevertheless do not yield satisfactory results, since painful sensations or a feeling of pressure may occur during erection. Hence, reduction-plasties should use techniques which shorten the erectile parts of the clitoris and reduce its size, while still maintaining sensitivity. Good cosmetic and tactile results may be achieved by means of selective excision of the corpora cavernosa and lateral clitoral excisions. Reconstruction of the labia minora out of clitoral shaft skin is combined with separate creation of a neo-preputium clitoridis.

Vaginal enlargement plasties have always been problematic, since shrinking particularly of the vaginal introitus, occurs in up to 25% of patients who undergo this operation. However, a sufficiently large pediculated perineal skin flap inserted into the "defect" of the posterior vaginal wall provides sufficient width of the vaginal introitus and canal.

Partial vaginal aplasia, with the vagina opening into a urogenital sinus near the bladder, calls for additional abdominal mobilisation. For psychological reasons, vaginal dilatations are not to be recommended. If necessary, a second vaginal enlargement plasty should instead be performed later; this may be carried out without problems before puberty. To avoid the disadvantage of a dry skin flap which does not assimilate to normal vaginal mucosa even after many years and with oestrogen treatment, mobilisation of the posterior vaginal wall with displacement of real vaginal mucosa towards the perineum can be carried out. However, one-stage reconstruction of clitoris, vulva and vagina during early childhood is preferable in every case, in order to avoid the psychological damage which can undoubtedly otherwise be caused. An exception is the late onset form of congenital adrenal hyperplasia.

Ruhr Univerity Bochum, Marienhospital, PO Box, 4690 Herne 1, FRG

Progress in Pediatric Surgery, Vol. 23
Ed. by L. Spitz et al.
© Springer-Verlag Berlin Heidelberg 1989

Zusammenfassung

Untersuchungen der letzten Jahre und Berichte über Spätergebnisse haben deutlich gemacht, daß der vaginale Orgasmus eher die Ausnahme als die Regel darstellt und daher eine Erhaltung der Klitoris-Sensibilität für die vita sexualis unerläßlich und immer anzustreben ist. Damit entfallen alle Korrektur-Operationen mit totaler Klitoridektomie, plastische Nachbildungen oder Klitorisverlagerungen mehr oder weniger unter die Symphyse. Auch wenn Plikationen und Versenkungen großer Klitorisschäfte unter den Mons pubis als sensibilitäts-erhaltende Maßnahmen eingestuft werden können, so befriedigen sie dennoch nicht, da sie im erigierten Zustand schmerzhafte Sensationen und Druckgefühl auslösen können. Es sind daher Reduktionsplastiken mit Verkürzung der erektilen Klitorisanteile unter Erhaltung der Glanssensibilität und eine Verkleinerung der Glans selbst anzustreben. Durch selektive Resektion der Corpora cavernosa und seitliche Exzisionen an der Glans sind gute kosmetische und taktile Ergebnisse zu erreichen. Die Rekonstruktion kleiner Labien aus Klitorisschafthaut wird mit einer separaten Neubildung eines Präputium clitoridis kombiniert.

Vaginalerweiterungs-Plastiken sind bisher hinsichtlich ihrer Spätergebnisse sehr problematisch geblieben, da Schrumpfungen, insbesondere des Introitus vaginae, in bis zu 25% beschrieben wurden. Durch einen ausreichend dimensionierten, dammwärts gestielten Hautlappen, der in einen durch dorsale Längsinzision entstandenen „Defekt" der Vaginalhinterwand einzubringen ist, gelingt es jedoch, eine ausreichende Weite von Vaginaleingang und Vaginalrohr zu erzielen.

Bei partieller Vaginalaplasie mit blasennaher Einmündung der Vagina in den Sinus urogenitalis ist eine zusätzliche Mobilisierung von abdominal her notwendig. Bougierungen der Vagina erscheinen aus psychologischen Gründen unangebracht. Es sollte, falls notwendig, eher auf eine zweite Vaginalerweiterungs-Plastik zurückgegriffen werden, was ohne Schwierigkeiten präpubertär möglich ist. Um die Nachteile des trockenen Hautlappens, der sich auch im Laufe von Jahren und unter Östrogeneinwirkung nicht der "Vaginalhaut" angleicht, zu beheben, kann eine Mobilisierung der Vaginalhinterwand mit dammwärtiger Verlagerung von eigentlicher Vaginalhaut erfolgen. Dennoch ist die einzeitige Frührekonstruktion von Klitoris, Vulva und Vagina wegen der unbestreitbaren, sonst möglichen, seelischen Schädigungen in jedem Fall vorzuziehen. Eine Ausnahme bildet die Spätform des AGS ("Late onset").

Résumé

Il ressort des études effectuées ces dernières années et des rapports récomment publiés que l'orgasme vaginal semble plutôt faire exception à la règle et qu'il est donc indispensable de préserver chaque fois que c'est possible la sensibilité du clitoris pour permettre une vie sexuelle normale. On renoncera donc à pratiquer toutes les interventions de correction nécessitant une clitoridectomie, les plasties ou déplacements du clitoris sous la symphyse. Même si les plications et les amar-rages de tissus du fourreau du clitoris de taille excessive sous le pubis peuvent être considérés comme une mesure ayant pour but de tenter de préserver la sensibilité, les résultats obtenus restent insuffisants car l'érection peut provoquer des sensations douloureuses et d'oppression. Il faudra donc envisager uniquement des plasties de réduction visant à raccourcir les parties érectiles du clitoris tout en conservant la sensibilité du gland dont on réduira aussi la taille. Une résection sélective du corps caverneux et des excisions latérales sur le gland donnent des résultats satisfaisants tant du point de vue esthétique que du point de vue tactile. On utilisera pour la reconstitution des petites lèvres la peau du fourreau du clitoris et on refera un prépuce séparément.

Les plasties destinées à dilater le vagin continuent à donner des résultats assez peu concluants et à poser des problèmes par la suite. En effet, on a rapporté jusqu'à 25% de rétrécissements ultérieurs, en particulier de l'introitus vaginae. En utilisant un lambeau pédiculé en direction du perinée et de taille suffisante qui sera placé dans une "dépression" de la paroi postérieure du vagin crée par une incision longitudinale dorsale, on obtiendra une largeur suffisante de l'entrée et du canal vaginal.

Dans les cas d'aplasie vaginale partielle avec abouchement du vagin près de la vessie dans le sinus urogénital, une mobilisation abdominale supplémentaire est requise. Pour des raisons psychologiques, il est déconseillé d'utiliser une bougie pour dilater. Il est préférable de procéder à une nouvelle plastie pour dilater le vagin, ce qui ne pose aucun problème avant la puberté. Pour parer aux inconvénients que pourrait poser la sécheresse du lambeau qui, au cours des années et en dépit de l'influence des oestrogènes ne s'assimilera pas à la muqueuse vaginale, on peut mobiliser la paroi postérieure du vagin en déplaçant la peau du vagin en direction du périnée. Quoi qu'il en soit, il faut toujours donner la préférence à une intervention en un seul temps pour reconstituer le clitoris, la vulve et le vagin pour éviter les troubles psychologiques qui ne manqueraient as de s'installer. Il existe une exception: la forme tardive de l'hyperplasie surrénale congénitale.

Introduction

Proper diagnosis and management of genital malformations are tasks which must be carried out with great responsibility, as undisturbed physical, psychological and sexual development depend on their results. Gender assignment and definitive genital correction should be carried out early enough for the child affected never to be aware of the genital abnormality or intersexuality. On the contrary: the small child must be allowed to identify itself with its physical gender (Knorr 1985; Prader 1980), similarly gender-specific upbringing by the parents can proceed emotionally undisturbed only if the external genitalia correspond to the gender role (Hecker 1985; Prader 1980). The time of gender identification is in the 3rd year of life (Hemminger 1982; Money and Schwarz 1977; Prader 1980; Schneider et al. 1968; Wilkins 1961). It follows that, in girls virilised antinatally by androgenic influences, the goal must be one-stage surgical correction of the genitalia before the second birthday is reached, aiming at an external appearance as close as possible to that of normal female genitalia, and normal ability for coitus and orgasm when sexual maturity is reached (Engert 1982).

This means:

1. Shortening of hypertrophied corpora cavernosa and reduction of the glans clitoridis while maintaining clitoral sensitivity
2. Reconstruction of a clitoral prepuce and labia minora and preservation of the urogenital chordee with its non-cornifying squamous epithelium
3. Enlargement of a narrow vaginal introitus and lengthening of a hypoplastic vaginal channel

In most cases virilisation of the external female genitalia is due to defective cortisol biosynthesis, which, in turn, is in 90% of patients due to a deficiency of 21-hydroxylase (Zachmann 1980). The degree of virilisation depends on the extent of this disturbance and is internationally classified into five stages, according to Prader (1980). Since the extent of visible, external virilisation indicates neither the level of the vaginal opening into the urogenital sinus, nor its relation to the vesical sphincter, nor the degree of vaginal hypoplasia, urethro-cysto-genitography and urethro-vaginoscopy are mandatory. With the exception of type I, in which only clitoral reduction is required, and type V, in which male gender identification and upbringing means, that vaginoplasty is contraindicated and an ovarectomy must be performed instead (Knorr 1985), further operative procedures depend exclusively on the level of vaginal opening and the degree of vaginal hypoplasia and aplasia.

Materials and Method

After implemenation in 1980 of a method which met the above mentioned criteria, and after a report of preliminary results in 1983, we now have results from a 5-year follow-up of 30 females of various ages (1–18 years; Engert 1982). The operative technique and its variations are described below:

Surgical Correction in Patients with a Low Vaginal Opening (Prader types I–III)

1. If no correction of a hypertrophied clitoris is necessary and if a vagina of sufficient width opens into the urogenital sinus at a low level, an inverted U-shaped (Stefan 1966) or M-shaped (Hecker 1985) pediculated skin flap originating from the perineum can be used for reconstruction of the posterior commissure.
2. If there is narrowing of the posterior part of the vagina, despite low opening of the vagina into the urogenital sinus, a long, inverted U-shaped pediculated skin flap hinged from the perineum has proved useful, starting from the tubera

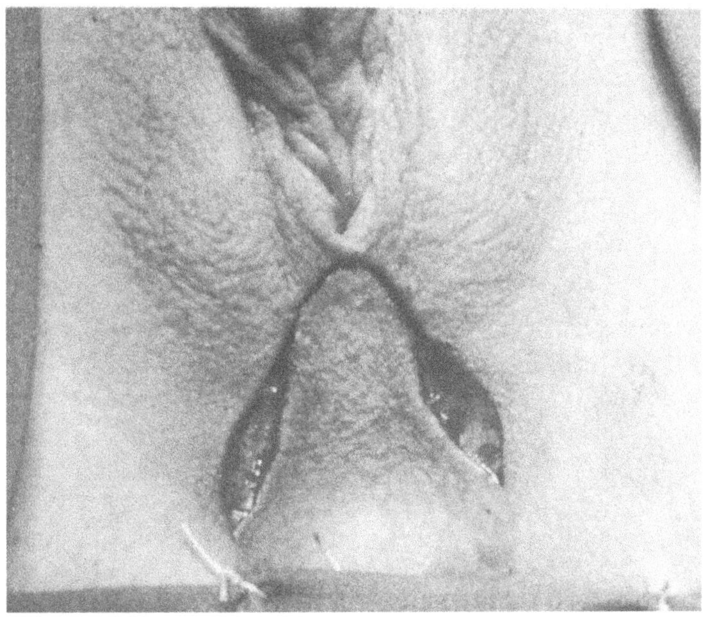

Fig. 1. Congenital adrenal hyperplasia, Prader type III. Incision of an inverted U-shaped pediculated skin flap hingeing from the perineum

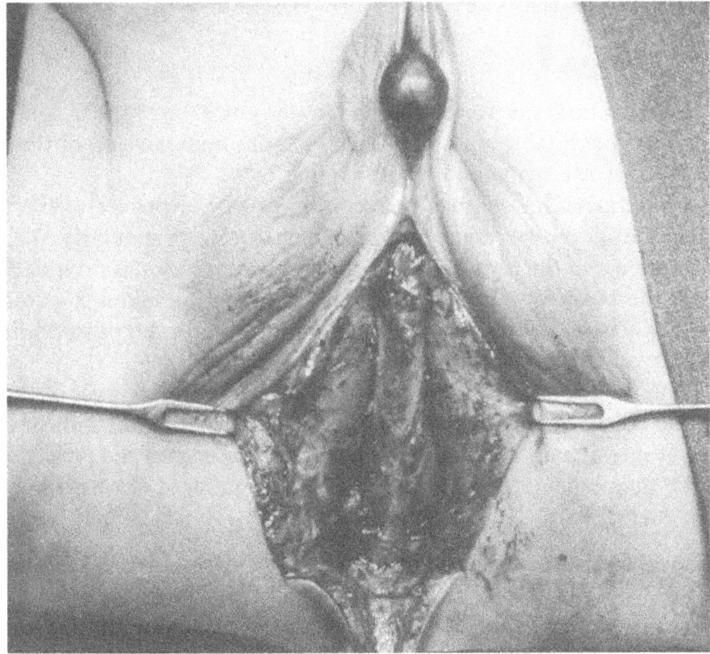

Fig. 2. Exposure of the urogenital sinus by longitudinal incision of the inner layer of the skin fold

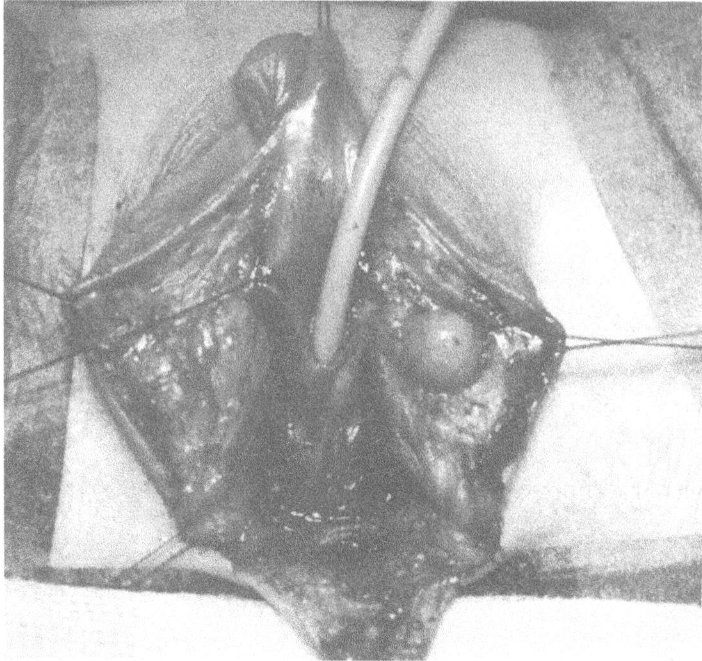

Fig. 3. Urogenital sinus partly exposed. The perineal muscles are visible

ischii on both sides and running into the entrance of the urogenital sinus (Fig. 1).
The urogenital sinus is opened by longitudinal incision of the inner layer up to
the narrowed vaginal introitus (Figs. 2, 3).

Preparation for surgery then continues with exposure of the posterior vaginal
wall and the perineal muscles (Figs. 4, 5), particularly the bulbocavernous
muscle and the urogenital diaphragm. Preparation is relatively straightforward
in the perineal region, particular care must be taken to avoid rectal injury as
the incision continues cranially. An intestinal tube passed into the rectum has
proved helpful for this.

The tength of the midline incision in the posterior wall of the vagina towards
the portio depends on the width of the vaginal lumen and/or the length of narrowed vagina; it is continued until the "defect" of the posterior wall is covered
by the pediculated skin flap, making a vagina of normal lumen (Fig. 6).

Surgical Correction in Patients with a High Vaginal Opening (Prader types IV, V)

A high vaginal opening near the bladder necessitates an abdomino-perineal procedure (Hecker 1985). In the first step, uterus and vagina are moved away from
the bladder and the rectum using an abdominal approach. Precise exposure of the

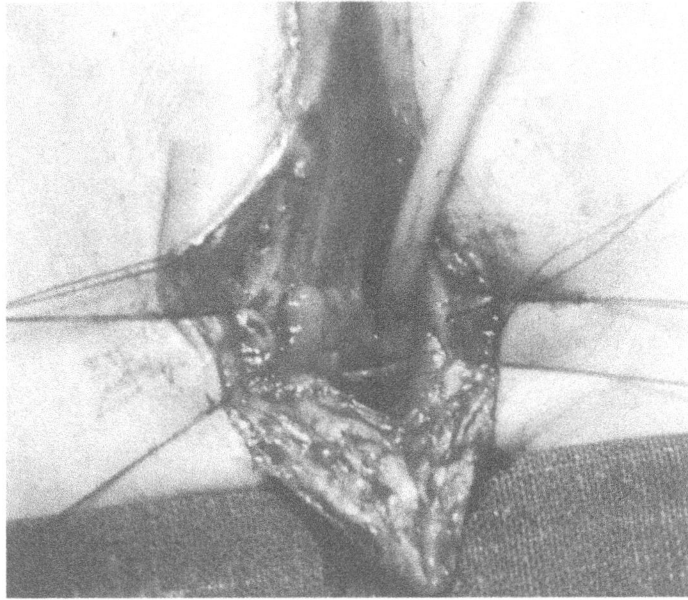

Fig. 4. Urogenital sinus entirely exposed. The posterior vaginal wall is prepared for operation

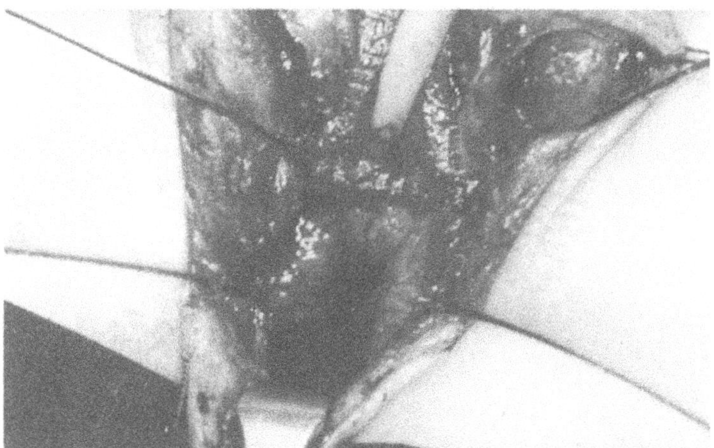

Fig. 5. Urethra and vagina after complete preparation. Since the vaginal lumen is of normal caliber, only the introitus and the posterior commissure need to be reconstructed

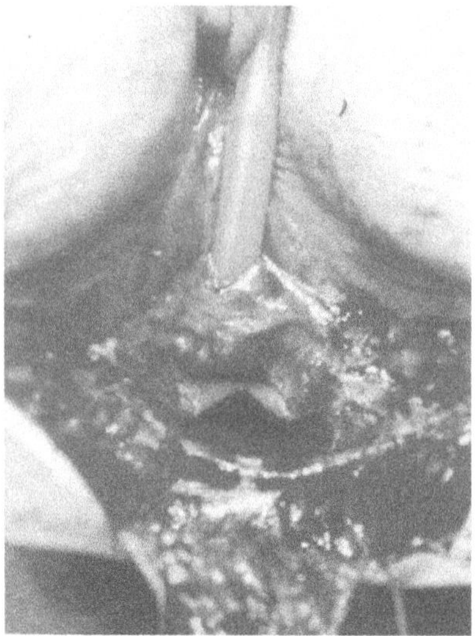

Fig. 6. Start of the incision in the posterior vaginal wall towards the portio

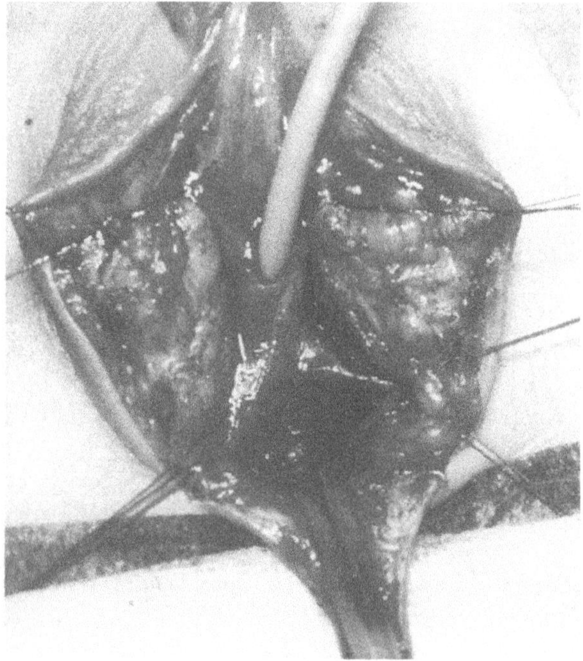

Fig. 7. Vaginal opening into the urogenital sinus pulled down by holding sutures following completion of the abdominal part of the operation

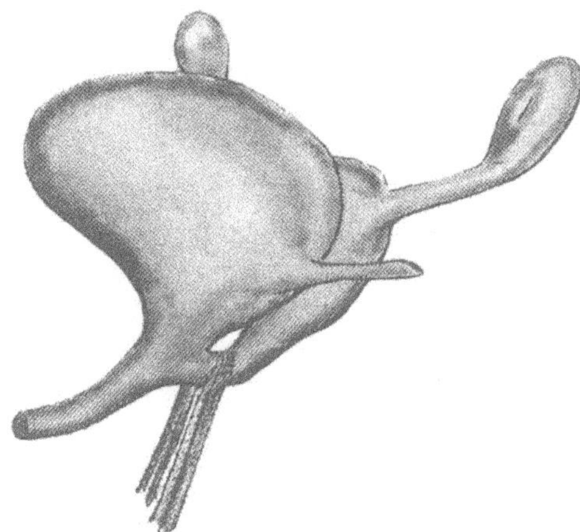

Fig. 8. High vaginal opening into the
sinus urogenitalis

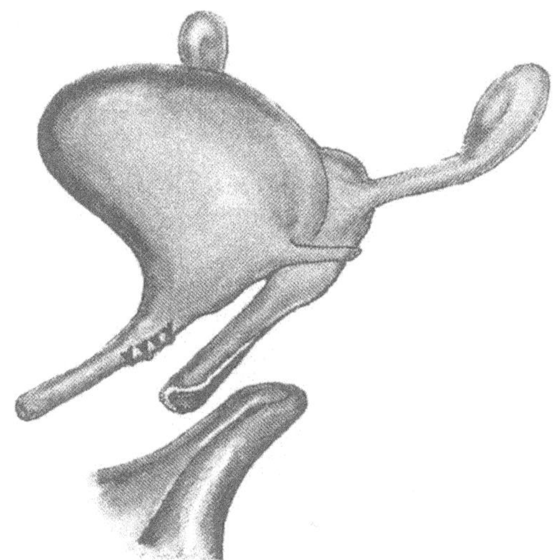

Fig. 9. Separation and closure of vaginal
opening into the sinus urogenitalis.
Dorsal vaginal incision towards to the
portio

high vaginal opening into the urogenital sinus is extremely important here. The
next step is carried out perineally, as outlined above; surgical correction is limited
by the extent of vaginal aplasia and the length of the pediculated perineal skin
flap. Following section and closure of the vaginal opening into the urogenital sinus
(Figs. 7–9), the vaginal canal is displaced caudally, dorsally incised to the portio,
and a oblique back-to-back anastomosis is carried out (Figs. 10, 11). Normally the
greater part of the new vaginal canal is created dorsally and distally to the pediculated perineal skin flap. If the vagina is short, the pediculated skin flap is closed
ventrally, forming a canal near the urethra.

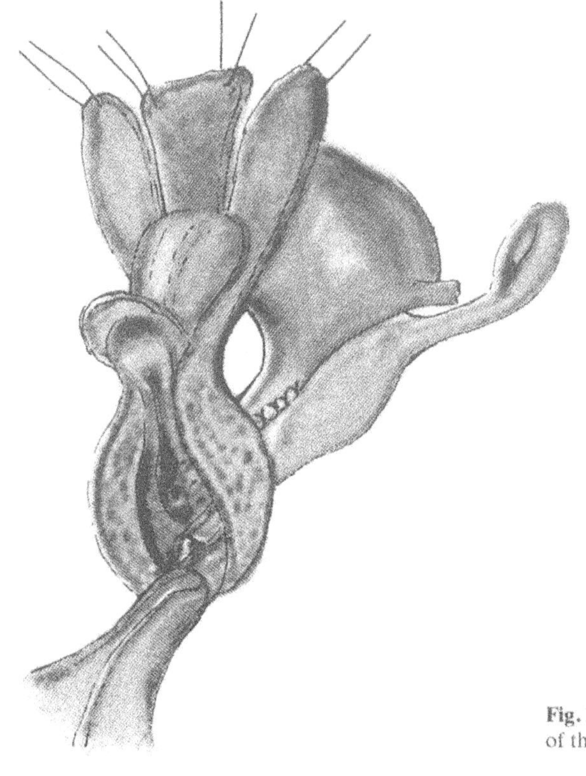

Fig. 10. Caudal displacement of the vaginal canal

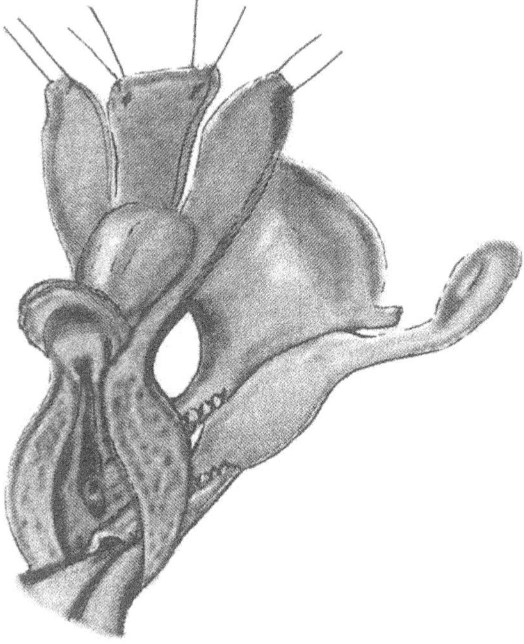

Fig. 11. Oblique back-to-back anastomosis with the pediculated skin flap

Surgical Correction of Vulva and Hypertrophied Clitoris

If there is clitoral hypertrophy requiring surgical correction, the procedures described above are combined with shortening of the corpora cavernosa, reduction of the glans clitoridis, and reconstruction of the clitoral prepuce and labia minora.

1. Starting at the tip of the U-shaped perineal skin flap, the glans clitoridis is circumcised, 5 mm of the inner preputial layer being preserved. The skin of the clitoral shaft is then entirely removed and the ligamentum arcuatum pubis exposed. The ligamentum suspensorium clitoridis is left intact; this is important for stabilisation of the clitoris. The superficial dorsal veins can be seen in the spongy superficial clitoral fascia. The usually impar deep dorsal vein of the clitoris, accompanied by the dorsal arteries and nerves of the clitoris, runs below the deep clitoral fascia and dorsal to the tunica albuginea. Since the position of the nerves unlike that of the arteries, is constant from patient to patient, it has been found useful to incise both the deep clitoral fascia and the tunica albuginea laterally on both sides and to separate the vessel-nerve bundle in toto from the corpora cavernosa in order to avoid injuries.
Following purse-string ligation of each corpus cavernosum separately to cut off the blood supplied by the deep clitoral arteries, most of the corpora cavernosa is removed (Figs. 12–14). However, at least 4 mm of the corpora cavernosa is left untouched near the glans, in order to maintain the stability of the glans

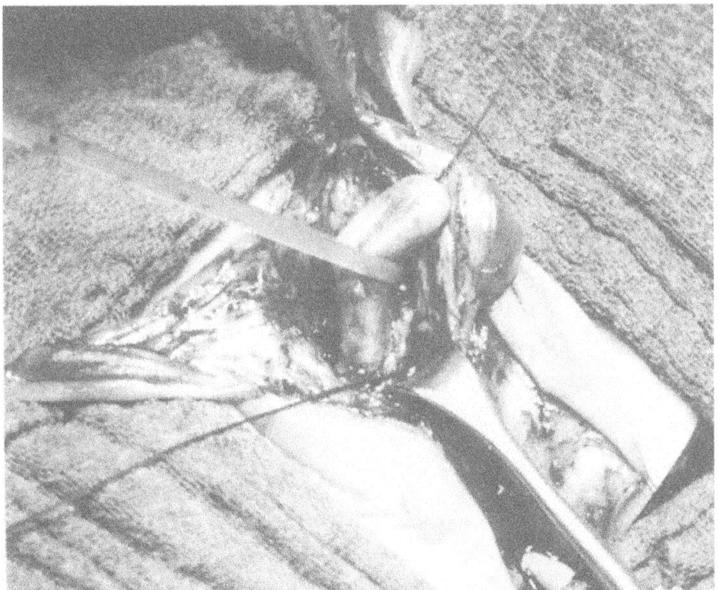

Fig. 12. Glans clitoridis, urogenital chordee and dorsal vessel-nerve bundle are separated. The corpora cavernosa are ligated to the length required

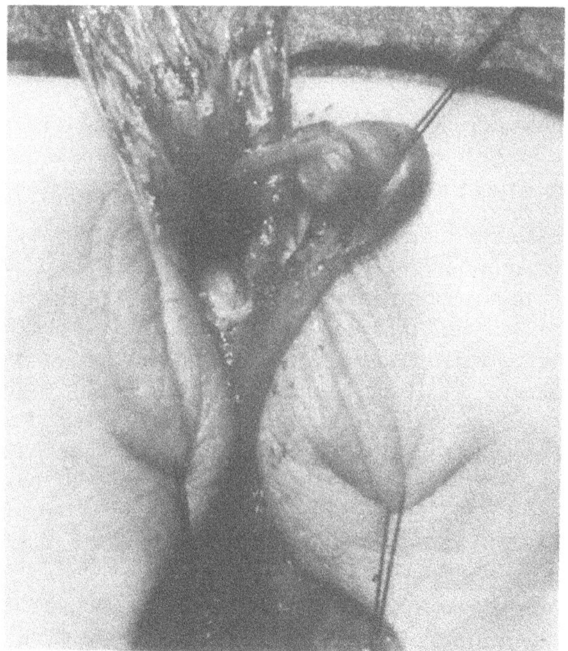

Fig. 13. Corpora cavernosa resected

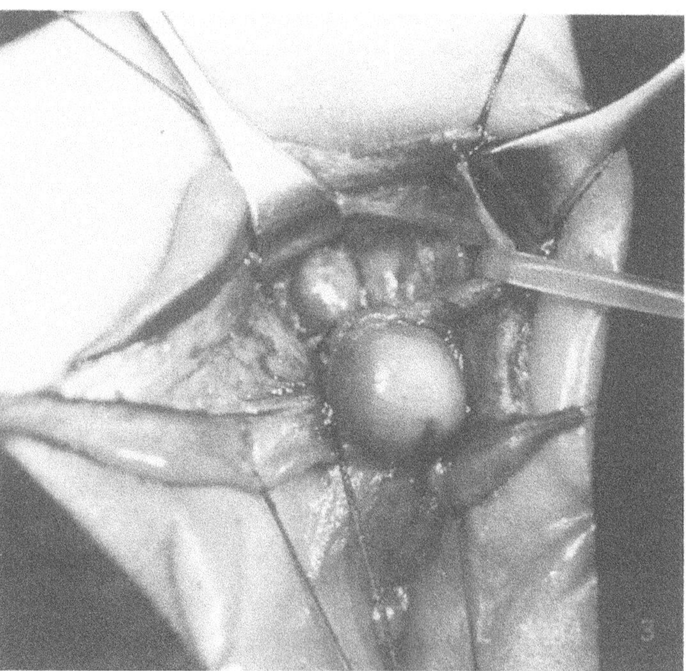

Fig. 14. The glans is refixed. It is too large, necessitating reduction by lateral excisions

and provide secure refixture to the remaining corpus clitoridis. Although, at the end of preparation, both the dorsal vessel-nerve bundle and the ventral urogenital chordee are preserved (the latter with its considerable blood supply to the glans and its non-cornifying squamous epithelium, so important for the vaginal introitus), it is advisable, if reduction of the glans by lateral excisions is necessary, to make this reduction dependant on the status of the blood supply to the glans, possibly postponing it until later.

2. Next, the preputial skin for covering the dorsal vessel-nerve bundle and glans clitoridis and for reconstructing the labia minora is prepared. This can be done using either one midline incision or – cosmetically more satisfying – two lateral incisions, leaving between them a median skin flap which alone is used for reconstruction of the prepuce. The doubled median skin flap, which covers the glans clitoridis entirely, is fixed laterally on both sides and caudally, and both lateral skin flaps, mimicking labia minora, are displaced towards the perineum. To improve their shape, the use of subcutaneous tie-up sutures is recommended. Surgical reduction or displacement of the labia majora towards the perineum is necessary in most cases.

Discussion

Contrary to the common view, we maintain that one-step surgical correction of clitorial hypertrophy and/or urogenital sinus with or without partial vaginal aplasia and reconstruction of the vulva can be carried out even in children under 2 years of age. With the help of a magnifying glass if necessary, it is always possible (a) to preserve the clitoral vessel-nerve bundle, essential to the sensitivity of the glans, and the ventral urogenital chordee, the non-cornifying squamous epithelium which is so important for the vaginal introitus, and (b) to reduce the corpora cavernosa to normal length. By means of lateral excisions, an overlarge glans clitoridis can be reduced to normal size without loss of sensitivity. The clitoris retrieves its stability postoperatively, and erections caused by the parasympathetic nerve fibers running along branches of the arteries have also been demonstrated. Division of the clitoral shaft skin into three, with reconstruction of the clitoral prepuce and labia minora, is another important step in the normalisation of the female external genitalia. Problems may arise with large clitoral shafts in that the blood supply to the shaft skin may be injured during preparation, so that the reconstruction of labia majora and clitoral prepuce have to be postponed to another session.

Vaginal orifice plasties and plastic surgery procedures for enlargeing or lengthening an aplastic vagina are still problematic in respect to late results regarding width of the vaginal introitus and channel. Use of a long, wide perineal skin flap originating from the region of the os ischii allows sufficient enlargement of the vaginal introitus and normalisation of the vaginal canal in most cases of partial vaginal aplasia. This has the advantage of better blood circulation than is present in the two laterally pediculated skin flaps described by Hecker (1985) and others and permits possible replacement of the distal aplastic part of the vagina in toto. This technique, however, is limited both by the extent of the vaginal aplasia and by the available length and width for the pediculated perineal skin flap. At a first operation, reconstruction of the vaginal canal can only establish a width of the vaginal lumen suitable to the patient's age at the time of operation, but attachment of the reconstructed vaginal canal to the perineum automatically causes the growth of the vagina to be oriented to the perineum. If the vaginal lumen should shrink, another enlargement plasty and reconstruction of a cosmetically more satisfying posterior commissure can be performed at puberty without changing the indication for primary surgical correction during early childhood. Since the transferred perineal skin, even with oestrogen treatment, will never become normal vaginal mucosa, the problem of the dry skin flap can be partly solved by means of mobilisation and displacement of vaginal mucosa towards the perineum in another operation. Although this results in shortening of the vaginal canal, normal length can be achieved by physiological bougienage later on.

References

Engert J (1982) Eine „physiologische" Korrektur des virilisierten weiblichen Genitale beim adrenogenitalen Syndrom. Paediatr Praxis 27:309–316

Hecker WC (1985) Operative Korrekturen des intersexuellen und des fehlgebildeten weiblichen Genitales. Springer, Berlin Heidelberg New York

Hemminger H (1982) Verhaltensbiologische Grundlagen der kindlichen Sexualentwicklung. In: Hellbrügge T (ed) Die Entwicklung der kindlichen Sexualität. Urban and Schwarzenberg, Munich

Hendren WH (1980) Urogenital sinus and anorectal malformation. J Paediatr Surg 15:628

Knorr D (1985) Pädiatrisch-endocrinologische Diagnostik bei Fehlbildung des weiblichen und bei intersexuellen Genitale. In: Hecker WC (ed) Operative Korrekturen des intersexuellen und des fehlgebildeten weiblichen Genitales. Springer, Berlin Heidelberg New York, pp 4–21

Money J, Schwarz M (1977) Dating, romantic and nonromantic friendships, and sexuality in 17 early treated adrenogenital females. In: Lee PA, Plotnick LP, Kowarski AA, Migeon CJ (eds) Congenital adrenal hyperplasia. University Park Press, Baltimore

Prader A (1980) Intersexualität. In: Bachmann KD, Everbeck H, Joppich G, Kleihauer G, Rossi E, Stalder GR (eds) Pädiatrie in Praxis und Klinik, vol 2. Fischer, Stuttgart, pp 14.80–14.88

Schneider KM, Becker JM, Krasner JH (1968) Surgical management of intersexuality in infancy and childhood. Ann Surg 168:255–261

Stefan H (1966) Chirurgische Behandlung des äußeren weiblichen Genitale beim weiblichen Pseudohermaphroditus. Z Kinderchir 3:249

Wilkins L (1961) Diagnosis and treatment of congenital virilizing and renal hyperplasia. Postgrad Med 29:31–39

Zachmann M (1980) Erkrankungen der Nebennierenrinde. In: Bachmann KD, Everbeck H, Joppich G, Kleihauer E, Rossi E, Stalder GR (eds) Pädiatrie in Praxis und Klinik. Fischer, Stuttgart, pp 14.89–14.103

Reconstruction of the Epispadiac Penis in Adolescents

C. R. J. Woodhouse

Summary

Now that reconstructive surgery has taken the exstrophy and epispadias patient beyond the stage of merely saving life and even preserving bladder function, it is essential that proper attention is paid to the penis. Careful surgery in early life may well give a good cosmetic appearance during the important years of schooling. It may also produce a penis with a satisfactory angle of erection for sexual intercourse. In those patients who are not so fortunate in infancy or who were born before the era of modern reconstructive surgery, careful assessment must be made at an appropriate time as the patient goes through puberty.

The commonest erectile deformity found in epispadias in adult life is tight dorsal chordee. Surgical correction is required. In some patients, adequate correction will be achieved by clearance of superficial pericorporeal scar tissue, possibly aided by Nesbit's procedure. For the remainder, formal correction of the chordee is required. This is best done by the insertion of a gusset of dura or other material to lengthen the concave side of the curve.

Zusammenfassung

Nachdem die plastische Chirurgie der Blasenexstrophie den Charakter einer ausschließlich lebensrettenden Maßnahme verloren hat und sogar die Erhaltung der Blasenfunktion möglich geworden ist, richtet sich das Interesse auf die Rekonstruktion des Penis, da diese Patienten eine normale Libido zeigen. Eine sorgfältige Operation im frühen Kindesalter kann durchaus ein gutes kosmetisches Ergebnis während der wichtigen Schuljahre geben. Es kann ebenso ein Erektionswinkel für einen normalen Sexualverkehr erreicht werden.

Bei jenen Patienten jedoch, bei denen im frühen Kindesalter eine weniger geglückte Operation durchgeführt worden war oder die vor der Ära der modernen plastischen Chirurgie geboren worden waren, muß eine sorgfältige Entscheidung zur richtigen Zeit getroffen werden, wenn sie in die Pubertät kommen. Die häufigste Form der Erektionsstörung beim Erwachsenen ist eine starke dorsale Krümmung, die die Operation erfordert. Bei manchen Fällen gibt eine Entfernung oberflächlicher pericorporaler Narbenzüge durch die Nesbit-Methode eine zufriedenstellende Korrektur. In den übrigen Fällen muß eine definitive operative

The Institute of Urology, University of London, 172 Shaftesbury Avenue, London WC2H 8JE, UK

Progress in Pediatric Surgery, Vol. 23
Ed. by L. Spitz et al.
© Springer-Verlag Berlin Heidelberg 1989

Korrektur der dorsalen Krümmung durchgeführt werden, was am besten durch eine Duraversteifung oder Implantation eines anderen Materials zum Ausgleich der Peniskrümmung erreicht wird.

Résumé

A l'heure actuelle, la chirugie plastique de l'extrophie de la vessie n'est plus uniquement une mesure de nécessité vitale et il est même possible de sauvegarder la fonction de la vessie. On peut donc maintenant très bien envisager la reconstitution du pénis car ces patients ont une libido normale. Une intervention pratiquée avec le plus grand soin dans la petite enfance pourra même donner des résultats assez satisfaisants du point de vue esthétique pour ne pas créer de difficultés pendant la période scolaire, ce qui est d'une grande importance. Il est possible aussi d'obtenir un angle d'érection suffisant pour des relations sexuelles normales. Dans le cas des patients qui dans leur petite enfance ont subi une intervention moins réussie ou qui sont nés avant l'avênement de la chirugie plastique moderne, il faudra soigneusement peser la décision de pratiquer une nouvelle intervention à l'âge de la puberté. Le trouble de l'érection le plus fréquent chez les adultes est une incurvation dorsale prononcée qui exige une intervention. Dans certains cas, on obtient une correction satisfaisante en pratiquant l'opération de NESBIT. Dans les autres cas, il faudra pratiquer une intervention de correction définitive de l'incurvation en raidissant ou en pratiquant une implantation pour compenser l'incurvation de la verge.

Introduction

In 1926 it was recorded that 50% of exstrophy patients were dead before the age of 10 (Mayo and Hendricks 1926). It is therefore hardly surprising that little attention was paid to the fate of the penis in reconstructing this major congenital abnormality. Over the last 40 years the results have improved considerably, and in a series of 101 cases followed into adult life, nine deaths were reported, only three of which could be directly attributed to the exstrophy and its management (Woodhouse et al. 1983). It is now generally expected that the exstrophy patient will grow up normally, attending normal schools, playing games, receiving higher education and undertaking a normal job (Jeffs 1978; Lattimer et al. 1979; Woodhouse et al. 1983).

Exstrophy patients have a normal libido. Now that growth into adult life is usual, it is reasonable to turn attention away from the immediate problems of survival and bladder closure towards reconstruction to allow normal intercourse. Even without reconstruction, the male with exstrophy can have a form of intercourse and there are several reports of paternity (Lattimer et al. 1976). However the epispadiac penis has an abnormal anatomy that is an integral part of the complex, though in some patients the deformity may have been aggravated by the reconstructive techniques for the bladder in infancy. The same abnormalities are found in epispadiac males with a split symphysis.

Typical Penile Anatomy in Exstrophy

The characteristic appearance of the adult exstrophy penis is shown in Fig. 1. It appears to be of approximately normal calibre but is clearly short and does not

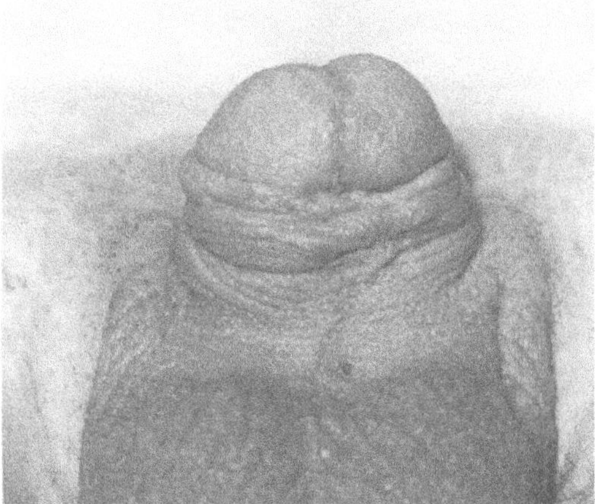

Fig. 1. Typical exstrophy penis

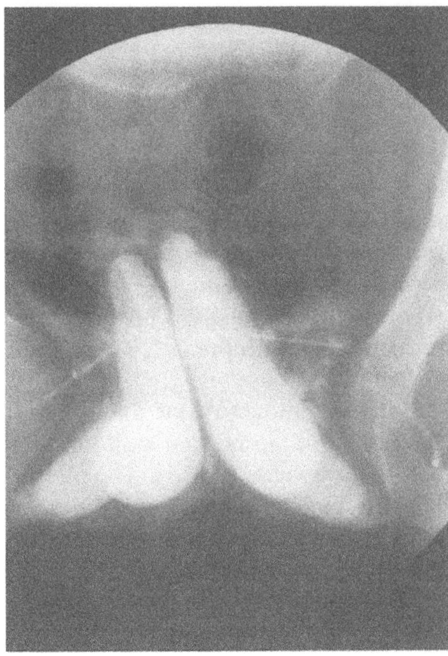

Fig. 2. Cavernosogram of exstrophy penis

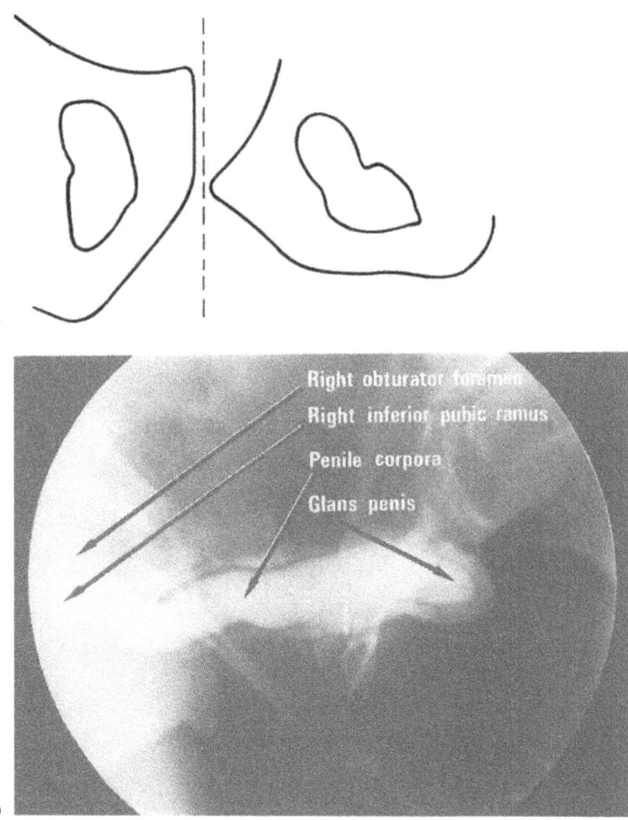

Fig. 3. a The normal pelvis *(left)* and the pelvis in exstrophy *(right).* **b** Oblique radiograph of a cavernosogram showing the anatomical position of the inferior pubic ramus in exstrophy

dangle. Investigation of the corpora by cavernosography and computerised axial tomography shows the reasons for this abnormality. The corpora are inherently short (Fig. 2). The shortness is further aggravated by corporeal length being taken up with reaching the midline from the widely separated inferior pubic rami. The corpora also have a sharp upward curve as they emerge from the perineum and this, combined with the lack of length in the exophytic portion, causes the lack of dangle (Woodhouse and Kellett 1984).

Oblique radiographs of the pelvis have shown that the inferior pubic ramus does not lie in the normal anatomical plane. Not only is the pelvis split but it is rotated downwards (Fig. 3). The inferior pubic ramus is thus parallel to the floor when the patient is standing (Woodhouse and Kellett 1984). This abnormality does not shorten the penis, but does have important implications for surgery designed to increase the length.

The superficial neurovascular bundle also lies in an abnormal position and its anatomy must be remembered in reconstructive operations at all ages. In the dis-

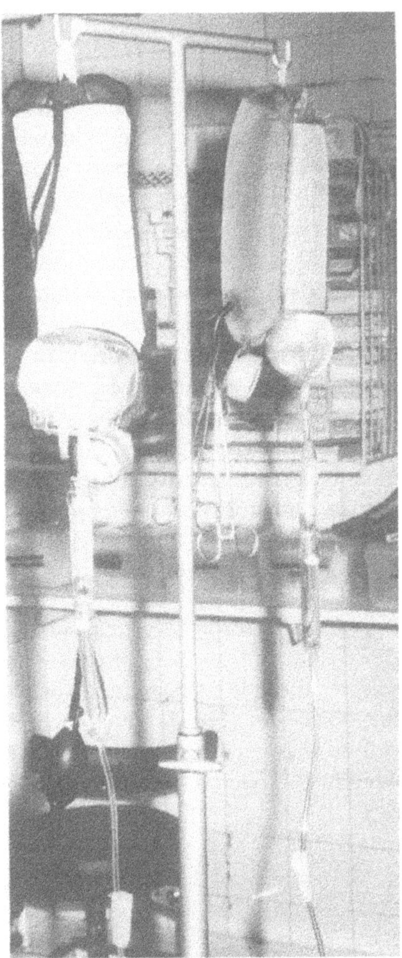

Fig. 4. System of infusion bags for cavernosogram

tal and middle portions of the corpora, the bundles are located in the 10 and 2 o'clock positions. As they pass proximally, they run more anteriorly to the 11 and 1 o'clock positions. They then merge into the cleft between the corpora and the pubic bone (Hurwitz et al. 1986).

It seems likely that this is the typical or "normal" anatomy of the penis in exstrophy and in split symphysis epispadias. It is seen to a greater or lesser degree in all patients. In particular, it is seen in split symphysis epispadiacs who have had no bladder-neck surgery and was also seen in a single patient with classical exstrophy who did not present until he was 44 (with carcinoma of the bladder), having previously had no surgery of any kind (Woodhouse and Kellett 1984). Excessive penile surgery in infancy can modify this anatomy and may, indeed, be responsible for some of the erectile deformities that are seen.

Erectile Deformities

Several types of erectile deformity are seen. The main deformity is a logical consequence of the typical anatomy already described. The others are almost certainly caused by excessive dissection in childhood. Unless the nature of the deformity is completely obvious, all cases should be investigated by preliminary cavernosography. The technique is modified from that described by Herzburg et al. (1981). In the epispadiac penis, there is no cross-circulation between the corpora, so that each side has to be injected separately. For this 120 ml 65% urografin is mixed with 250 ml physiological saline. The infusion is made from two bags through separate 19-gauge butterfly needles. A pressure of 300 mm Hg is generated by infusion bags (Fig. 4). The procedure can usually be carried out under sedation with intravenously administered diazepam, though occasionally a general anaesthetic is necessary for rather anxious patients.

The following description of erectile deformities is based on investigation of 20 patients (Woodhouse 1986). It lacks full supporting evidence from other sources, but the patterns have been consistent throughout the investigation and in patients seen subsequently. Similar deformities have been reported by Brzezinski et al. (1986) in adolescent patients.

Type 1 − Dorsal Chordee. This is the commonest erectile deformity, seen in three-quarters of the patients. The characteristic short corpora are of normal calibre; there is a sharp dorsal curvature, often of 90°, as the corpora emerge from the perineum (Fig. 5). The erect penis is pressed tightly against the abdominal wall so that vaginal penetration is impossible. This erectile deformity is that which would be expected on the basis of the typical anatomy.

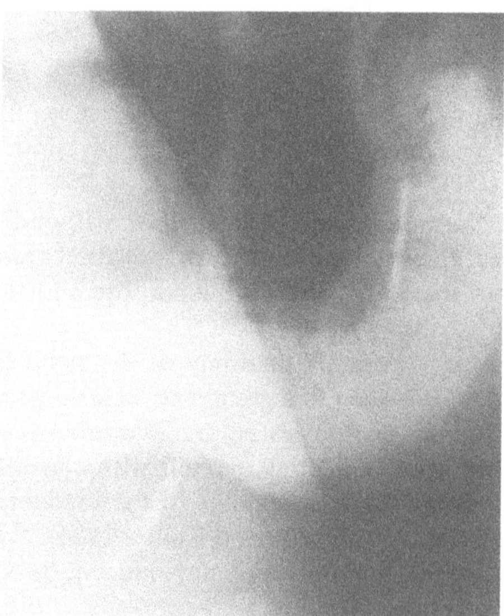

Fig. 5. Lateral radiograph of a cavernosogram showing nearly 90° of dorsal chordee

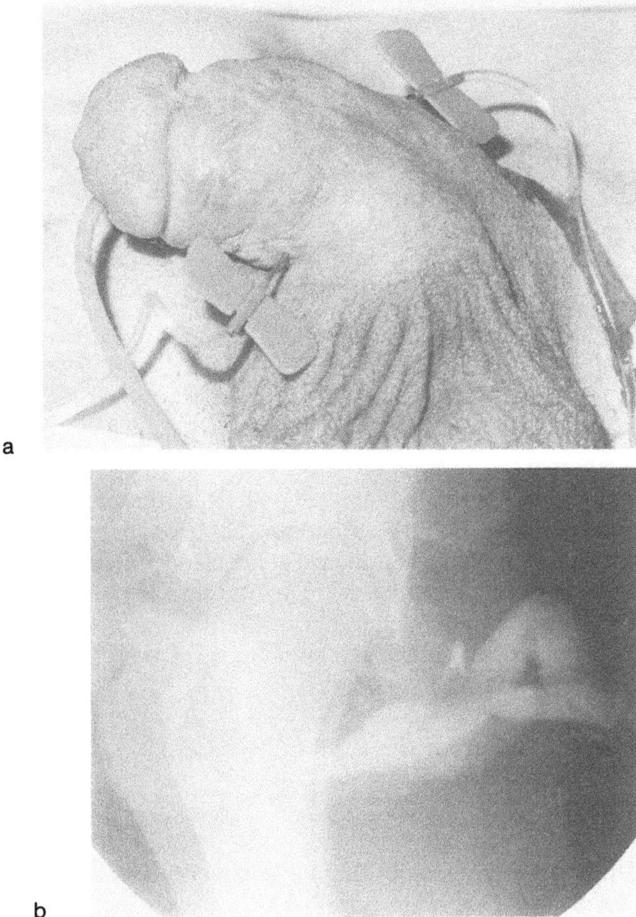

Fig. 6. a Artificial erection showing dorsal chordee and sharp lateral deviation. **b** Lateral radiograph of the same case, showing that the right corpus is rudimentary and causes "bowstringing" of the normal left corpus

Type 2 — Lateral Deviation. This abnormality was seen in 2 of 20 patients. In the flaccid state, the penis looks no different from any other epispadiac penis. When erect, there is dorsal chordee and sharp lateral deviation so that the penis points at the hip joint. It occurs because one corpus is normal, while the other is rudimentary. On erection, the rudimentary corpus fails to expand and pulls the normal corpus over to that side (Fig. 6). It seems likely that the rudimentary corpus has been damaged during dissection at previous surgery.

Type 3 — Micro-erection. This abnormality was seen in 3 of 20 patients. The flaccid penis also has the typical epispadiac appearance, although it is usually higher

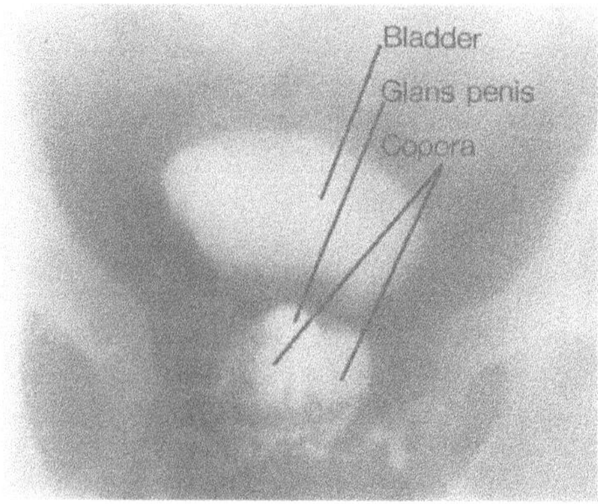

Fig. 7. Anterior-posterior radiograph of a cavernosogram/cystogram showing rudimentary development of both corpora. There is no deep portion and no attachment to the inferior pubic rami

on the mons pubis. On erection, the expansion is minimal. Cavernosography shows that the corpora are short and have no deep portion and thus no connection with the inferior pubic rami (Fig. 7). This abnormality, too, must surely be due to excessive dissection. A further case has been seen in an epispadiac who had had 12 operations to obtain continence at the bladder neck, in the course of which his penis had completely disappeared. The urethra emerged through a fold in the scrotum. On palpation under general anaesthetic it was possible to feel a very rudimentary left corpus deep in the perineum but there was nothing to feel on the right.

Corrective Surgery

Timing

The erectile deformities that have been described were found in patients who are now adults. They were born between the second World War and 1966. The techniques of reconstruction have changed considerably since then, and children born now may not require penile reconstruction in adulthood (Mesrobian et al. 1986). In some patients, the need for dorsal chordee correction is anticipated by the insertion of ellipses of dura in the dorsum of the penis during the initial reconstruction (P. G. Ransley, personal communication 1986), though it remains to be seen whether the correction achieved will be maintained in adulthood.

There can be no doubt that the penis should be made as normal as possible in infancy. The appearance and function of the penis is of paramount concern to the adolescent with exstrophy (Feinberg et al. 1974).

If the boy arrives at puberty with an erectile deformity, the timing of correction becomes very difficult, especially if the question of schooling is considered. It is preferable to make the correction when the boy has had some practical experience of intercourse. He can thus appreciate his own deficiency and the objectives to be achieved. However, surgery should not be delayed until several embarrassing failures have damaged his ego.

Procedures

In patients with the common deformity of dorsal chordee, there are two components that require correction: the overall length of the visible portion of the penis and the angle. Both are important, but if it is the case that the corpora are deficient in overall length rather than merely *apparently* short because of the divarication of the pelvic bones, improvement in this aspect is likely to be less successful.

Lengthening Procedures

Several procedures have been described for the lengthening of the epispadiac penis. In some patients, probably because the corpora have become "concertina-ed" by the urethral plate, scar tissue and poor skin, extensive dissection and covering with new skin will produce considerable lengthening. Good results have been reported by this procedure alone in the younger patient (Hendren 1979). However, such simple procedures have not proved effective in the adolescent group in the author's experience. It may be that by this stage in life, secondary and irreversible changes have occurred in the corpora.

It has been pointed out that if the divarication of the pelvic bones is 3 cm or less, the penis is apparently longer than if it is 4 cm or more (Schillinger and Wiley 1984). However, Johnston (1974) found that bringing the pelvic bones into apposition by posterior osteotomy did not increase the penile length. Whatever the case may be in children, osteotomy does not seem a very attractive prospect in the adolescent. Those adolescents who had a pelvic osteotomy as part of their primary repair in infancy have not retained the apposition of the pubis into adult life.

If it is correct that the inferior pubic ramus is parallel with the floor when the patient is standing (Woodhouse and Kellett 1984), dissection of the corpora off the pubis will not help if it is continued posterior to the junction with the inferior pubic ramus. Kelley and Eraklis (1971) described complete detachment of the corpora from the inferior pubic ramus and drawing them forward, presumably on the vessels from Alcock's canal. The report covered four cases and there was no long-term follow-up. This would seem rather a hazardous procedure that could lead to devascularization of one or both corpora. Indeed, it is possible that excessive dissection of this sort in children is the cause of the erectile deformity types 2 and 3.

Thus, it seems that in adolescents there is no worthwhile procedure for lengthening the visible portion of the epispadiac penis alone. Complete stripping of the pericorporeal scar tissue and the urethral plate forms a part of the surgery designed to correct chordee and may provide some lengthening.

Chordee Correction

The need for chordee correction must be carefully assessed. In some cases the patient's description alone provides an obvious enough indication. Where there is doubt, a cavernosogram should be performed and the surgeon should be present at the examination to assess the problem for himself. The present generation of

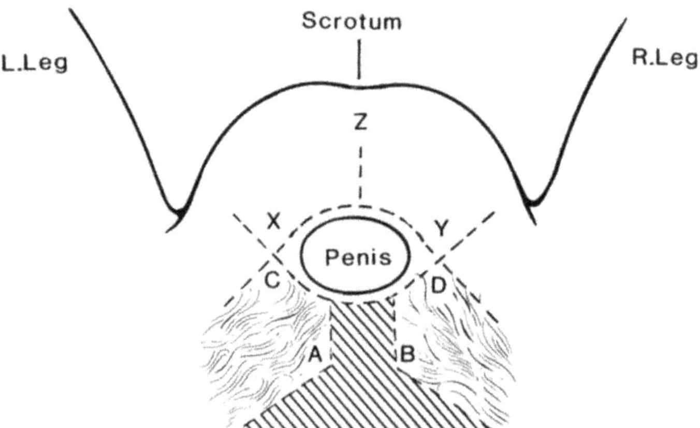

Fig. 8. Commonly used incision for exstrophy phalloplasty. The *shaded area* is scarred and will be excised

DORSUM OF EPISPADIAC PENIS

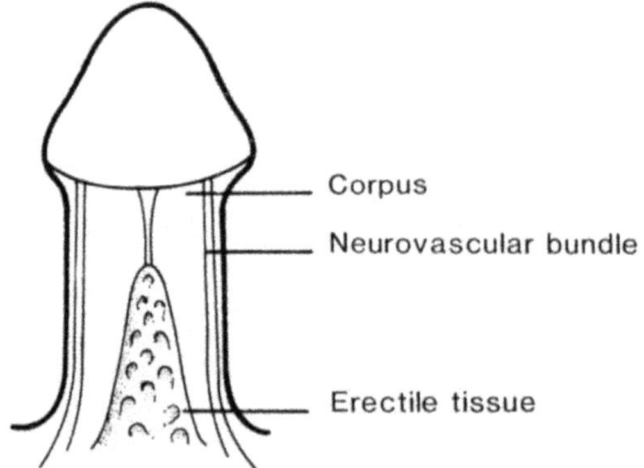

Fig. 9. Extra-corporeal erectile tissue

adolescents and young adults appear, in the author's experience, very commonly to require chordee correction. Others have not found this to be the case (Mesrobian et al. 1986), and it may be that better management of the penis in infancy may lessen the need for this type of surgery in later life.

All the operations described are done under general anaesthetic with the patient flat on the table. Whatever the preoperative investigation has been, frequent intra-operative artificial erection is essential. The technique is that already described for cavernosography, though without the contrast medium.

There is no standard incision because no two patients are the same. Incisions are made appropriate to the skin flaps that are going to be required for closure. In particular, the need for rotation of hair-bearing skin from the groins to the midline must be considered. A commonly used incision is shown in Fig. 8.

The dissection of the corpora is started at their apparent junction with the body of the pubis. It is continued until the corpora have been separated from the bone down to the anterior end of the inferior pubic ramus. The urethra − assuming that it is lying on the dorsum of the penis − is completely mobilised off the corpora. There is a triangle of extra-corporeal erectile tissue surrounding the urethral plate in this area (Fig. 9); its mobilisation causes troublesome bleeding. In about 50% of cases, the urethra is clearly too short and needs to be transected. The corpora are completely stripped of all apparent fibrous tissue on the dorsum and on either side, thus separating the corpora from each other through to the ventrum. At this stage, a further artificial erection is made. In only 1 of 15 of the author's cases (Woodhouse 1986) but in 4 of 8 cases reported by Brzezinski and co-workers (Brzezinski et al. 1986) did it transpire that this dissection was sufficient to correct the chordee.

If the chordee does persist, a formal correction is required. A variety of techniques has been described. Theoretically, there are two basic principles for the straightening of a curve in a parallel-sided cylinder: lengthening the concave side or shortening the convex side. In the case of the penis which is already too short, further shortening, as in Nesbit's procedure (Frank et al. 1981), is unsatisfactory. Nevertheless, Nesbit's procedure remains an option for chordee correction. Good results have been reported in a small number of cases (Brzezinski et al. 1986; Woodhouse 1986). It is particularly indicated where the amount of correction required is small, so that there will be little shortening of the penis overall, and where the patient is unwilling to accept the complications that can follow the more radical procedures.

To lengthen the concave side of the corpora, a transverse incision is made on the dorsum of the penis at the point of greatest curvature. The incision must encompass at least five-eighths of the circumference and be deep enough to divide the trabeculations of the corpora albuginea. When the penis is straightened out, there is an elliptical defect in the tunica albuginea to be filled with suitable material.

Several autologous and synthetic materials have been used. Most have been adapted from procedures for the correction of Peyronie's disease. Materials include fat (Lowsley and Boyce 1950), aponeurosis (Bruschini and Mitre 1979), tunica vaginalis, (Das 1980), Dacron (Lowe et al. 1982), Dexon mesh (Bazeed et al. 1983), skin (Horton and Devine 1973) and lyophilised human dura mater (Woodhouse 1986). Of these, only skin and dura have been widely used in the correction of chordee in adult exstrophy patients (Horton and Devine 1973; Brzezinski et al. 1986; Woodhouse 1986). Skin has been used principally in younger patients.

Technique of Dural Phalloplasty. The initial steps of the dissection are the same whatever technique of chordee correction is ultimately used. If the mid-operation artificial erection shows that a formal correction is required, the sheet of dura (B. Braun, Melsungen, FRG) to be used is removed from its packet and soaked in saline while the other preparations are made. An ellipse of tinfoil is prepared

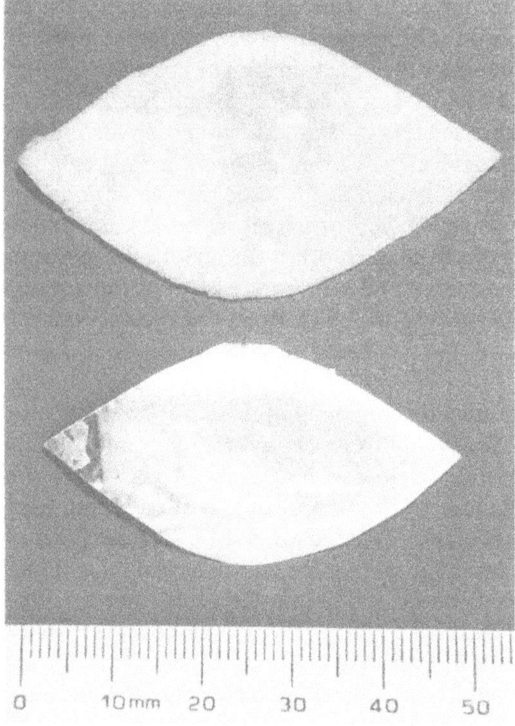

Fig. 10. Tinfoil template and dural ellipse

(Fig. 10), of which the long axis is determined by the circumference of the corpus and the short axis by the amount of correction that is required. The short axis normally measures about 3 cm. It is important to be generous to allow for increase in size during erection. An ellipse of dura is then cut using the tinfoil as a template. The dural ellipse is made larger than the tinfoil to allow for suturing (Fig. 10).

The procedure is then the same for each corpus. The transverse incision is made. It is surprising how deep this incision has to be to divide the trabeculations of the tunica albuginea; at times it seems as though the entire corpus is being transected. The dura is sutured into the defect using continuous 2/0 Dexon. A further artificial erection is then made to check that the correction is adequate.

Any further skin flaps are mobilised and closed with Dexon, employing continuous suction drainage. If the incision was made as in Fig. 8, the closure will be similar to that shown in Fig. 11. Antibiotic cover is given routinely, using a broad spectrum such as ampicillin and metronidazole. It is continued for 5 days.

Complications of Dural Phalloplasty. In 13 cases, only one serious complication has been encountered, which was an extensive wound infection in one patient before the policy of routine administration of prophylactic antibiotics was instigated. Fortunately, the infection settled with antibiotic treatment and the ultimate out-

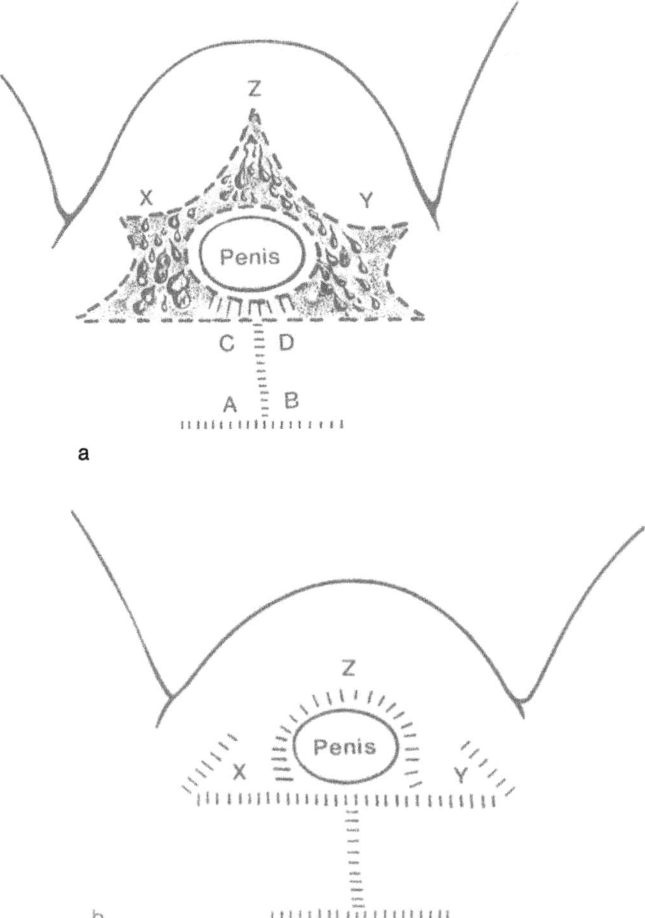

Fig. 11a, b. Closure, assuming incisions as shown in Fig. 8. **a** First stage, **b** second stage

come was satisfactory. A further patient was impotent for 3 months after the operation but eventually recovered spontaneously.

The Urethra in Chordee Correction. When the urethra is on the dorsum of the penis, it is normally too short to allow full chordee correction. It will thus require division. If a graft of dura or skin is used, it is better to leave urethroplasty until a second operation (Brzezinski et al. 1986). However, if there is no graft, ure-throplasty can be performed in the same operation, or, in some cases, the old urethra may even be preserved.

The practice of transposing the urethra to the ventrum of the penis (R.T. Turner-Warwick, personal communication, 1983) is to be applauded both for its cosmetic advantage and for the correction of chordee. In cases of dural phal-loplasty with a dorsal urethra it is helpful, when transecting the urethra, to make the proximal end long enough to pass between the corpora and be brought out as a cutaneous fistula on the ventrum.

Urethroplasty in the adult epispadiac penis is difficult. In designing the skin flaps at the original chordee correction, it is important to bear in mind the positioning of skin suitable for later reconstruction. A good deal of imagination is required to devise systems of reconstruction and in the 13 cases reported above, 6 patients have undergone urethroplasty, requiring 15 revision procedures (Woodhouse 1986). Patients who have a urinary diversion will sometimes elect to keep a proximal seminal fistula rather than risk the complications of reconstruction.

Results of Chordee Correction. It seems likely that careful chordee correction in infancy would be successful in the long term. Of 56 cases, 53% assessed in adult life were judged to have been cosmetically successful in the Mayo Clinic series (Mesrobian et al. 1986). Nonetheless, great caution must be exercised in the corporeal dissection in infancy to avoid damaging the blood supply (Ransley 1986).

Chordee correction with an angle of dependency of better than 45° has been reported in 7 of 8 patients, 4 of whom had had a dermal graft phalloplasty (Brzezinski et al. 1986). The results of dural phalloplasty in the author's own series of older patients are not quite so good. In 8 of 12 patients the result was satisfactory at the first attempt and in one patient at a second attempt. In 1 patient the correction appeared satisfactory but a further chordee appeared distal to the site of the first repair 18 months later; this was corrected by a further dural phalloplasty. In 2 patients the result was unsatisfactory and they are awaiting further surgery (Woodhouse 1986). A typical example of erection before and after dural phalloplasty is shown in Fig. 12.

The causes of failure are not clear. With the 1 exception mentioned above, the failure was apparent as soon as the wounds had healed and the first erections occurred. In the successful cases, the angle of erection has been maintained at follow-up from 2 to 5 years in six cases of dural phalloplasty. It may be that the incision of the corpora heals across, in spite of the presence of the graft. Correction by Nesbit's procedure, in the small number of cases reported, has been uniformly successful.

Following surgery, patients in whom the operation has been successful are able to have satisfactory intercourse. There is marginal lengthening of the penis, which should really be regarded as a beneficial side effect of the procedure. Limited vaginal penetration is possible.

Surgery for Types 2 and 3 Erectile Deformity

Type 2. In the first case encountered in which one rudimentary corpus was causing "bowstringing" of the normal one, the rudimentary corpus was divided. This procedure was not satisfactory, as it became apparent that two corpora are needed for a stable erection, each to support the other as in the gables of a house. In subsequent cases, the lateral and dorsal curvature have been corrected by large ellipses of dura in a similar manner to that described above. The results have been

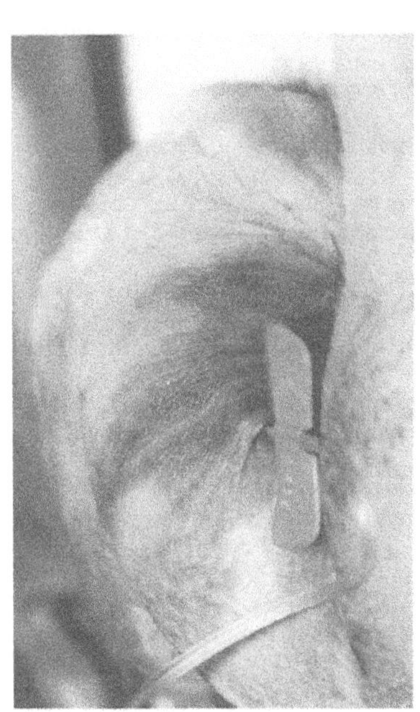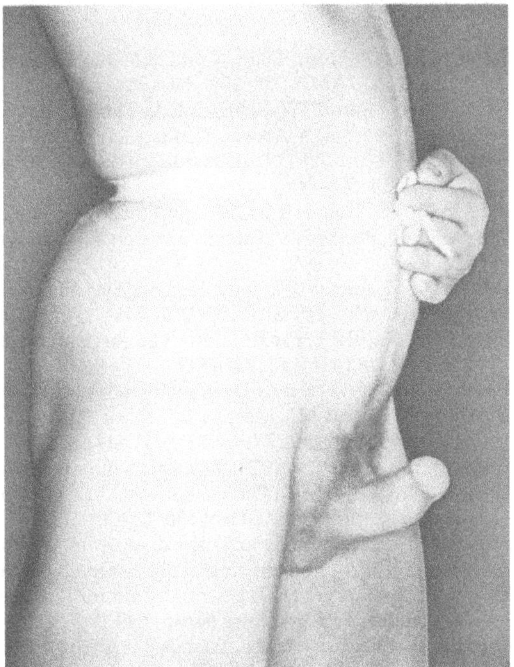

a   b

Fig. 12. a Artificial erection before and **b** natural erection after dural phalloplasty

satisfactory. This is a rare complication of exstrophy and epispadias and requires careful preliminary assessment including a cavernosogram.

Type 3. There have been no reports of surgery for this rare deformity. In the present state of the art, it is probably inoperable. The corpora are extremely rudimentary and have no apparent connection with the inferior pubic ramus. It therefore seems likely that they do not receive a blood or nerve supply through the Alcock's canal. Any surgery would be likely to damage what little collateral supply they have from the superficial vessels, thus making the situation worse.

Addendum. It has recently been reported that the sterilisation procedures for human dura are not adequate to inactivate the Creutzfeld-Jacob agent. A case has been reported of a 28-year-old woman who died of Creutzfeld-Jacob disease 22 months after receiving a dural graft (Anonymous 1987). Although some preparations of dura are processed in different ways, the American Food and Drug Administration considers that all the preparations carry a risk of transmitting this disease. In the light of this finding, the author thinks it would be preferable to use this technique with material from the patient such as rectal sheath or tunica vaginalis rather than dura.

References

Anonymous (1987) Up Date: Creutzfeld-Jacob disease in a patient receiving a cadaveric dura mater graft. JAMA 258:309–310 (editorial)

Bazeed MA, Thuroff JW, Schmidt RA, Tanagho EA (1983) New surgical procedure for management of Peyronie's disease. Urology 21:501–504

Bruschini H, Mitre AI (1979) Peyronie's disease: surgical treatment with muscular aponeurosis. Urology 13:505–506

Brzezinski AE, Homsy YL, Laberge I (1986) Orthoplasty in epispadias. J Urol 136:259–261

Das S (1980) Peyronie's disease: excision and autografting with tunica vaginalis. J Urol 124:818–819

Feinberg T, Lattimer JK, Jeter K, Langford W, Beck L (1974) Questions that worry children with exstrophy. Pediatrics 53:242–246

Frank JD, Mor SB, Pryor JP (1981) The surgical correction of erectile deformities of the penis of 100 men. Br J Urol 53:645–648

Hendren WH (1979) Penile lengthening after previous repair of epispadias. J Urol 121:527–534

Herzburg Z, Kellett MJ, Morgan RJ, Pryor JP (1981) Method, indications and results of corpus cavernosography. Br J Urol 53:641–644

Horton CE, Devine CJ (1973) Peyronie's disease. Plast Reconstr Surg 52:503–510

Hurwitz RS, Woodhouse CRJ, Ransley PG (1986) The anatomical course of the neurovascular bundles in epispadias. J Urol 136:68–70

Jeffs RD (1978) Exstrophy and cloacal exstrophy. Urol Clin North Am 5:127–140

Johnston JH (1974) Lengthening of the congenital or acquired short penis. Br J Urol 46:685–687

Kelley JH, Eraklis AJ (1971) A procedure for lengthening the phallus in boys with exstrophy of the bladder. J Pediatr Surg 6:645–649

Lattimer JK, Macfarlane MT, Pucher PJ (1976) Male exstrophy patients: a preliminary report on the reproductive capability. Trans Am Assoc Genitourinary Surg 70:42–46

Lattimer JK, Hensle TW, Macfarlane MT, Beale L, Braun E, Eposito Y (1979) The exstrophy support team: a new concept in the care of the exstrophy patient. J Urol 121:472–473

Lowe DH, Ho PC, Parsons CL, Schmidt JD (1982) Surgical treatment of Peyronie's disease with dacron graft. Urology 19:609–610

Lowsley OS, Boyce WM (1950) Further experiences with an operation for the cure of Peyronie's disease. J Urol 63:888–892

Mesrobian H-GJ, Kelalis PP, Kramer SA (1986) Long-term follow-up of cosmetic appearance and genital function in boys with exstrophy: review of 53 patients. J Urol 136:256–258

Ransley PG (1986) Exstrophy/epispadias: discussion. J Urol 136:262–263

Schillinger JF, Wiley MJ (1984) Bladder exstrophy penile lengthening procedure. Urology 24:434–437

Woodhouse CRJ (1986) The management of erectile deformity in adults with exstrophy and epispadias. J Urol 135:932–935

Woodhouse CRJ, Kellett MJ (1984) Anatomy of the penis and its deformities in exstrophy and epispadias. J Urol 132:1122–1124

Woodhouse CRJ, Ransley PG, Williams DI (1983) The patient with exstrophy in adult life. Br J Urol 55:632–635

One-Stage Preputial Pedicle Flap Repair for Hypospadias: Experience with 100 Patients

P. Frey[1] and A. Bianchi[2]

Summary

Between 1980 and 1986, 224 patients underwent one-stage hypospadias repair, of whom 100 were operated on using a modification of the Asopa technique. This technique, in which a vascularised preputial pedicle flap is rotated ventrally in order to reconstruct a neo-urethra as well as to cover the ventral skin defect, is described. The post-operative results are discussed. Fistula formation was the most common complication, but was easily correctable.

Zusammenfassung

Von 1980–1986 wurden 224 Patienten mit Hypospadie einer einzeitigen Korrektur unterzogen, von denen 100 nach einer modifizierten Asopa-Methode operiert wurden. Diese Methode, bei der ein vaskularisierter, gestielter Präputiallappen nach ventral zur Konstruktion der Neourethra und zur Deckung des ventralen Hautdefektes rotiert wird, wird beschrieben. Die postoperativen Ergebnisse werden diskutiert. Fistelbildung war die häufigste, jedoch leicht zu korrigierende Komplikation.

Résumé

Entre 1980 et 1986 nous avons pratiqué une intervention de correction en un temps dans le cas de 224 patients présentant un hypospadias. 100 de ces patients ont été opérés d'après la méthode Asopa, modifiée. Elle consiste à effectuer la rotation en direction ventrale d'un lambeau pédonculé et vascularisé du prépuce pour reconstituer l'urètre et recouvrir le défaut de la peau ventrale. Les auteurs discutent les résultats postopératoires. La complication la plus fréquente est la formation d'une fistule mais elle est facile à traiter.

---

[1] Department of Neonatal Surgery, St. Mary's Hospital, Whitworth Park, Manchester M13 OJH, United Kingdom. *Current address:* Kinderchirurgische Klinik, Universitäts Kinderspital Basel, Römergasse 8, CH-4005 Basel, Switzerland
[2] Department of Paediatric Surgery, Royal Manchester Children's Hospital, Hospital Road, Pendlebury, Manchester, M27 IHA, United Kingdom

Progress in Pediatric Surgery, Vol. 23
Ed. by L. Spitz et al.
© Springer-Verlag Berlin Heidelberg 1989

Introduction

For decades, hypospadias have been corrected in at least two stages (Ombrédanne 1923; Byars 1950; Cecil 1952; Brown 1953; Culp 1959; Fugua and Belt 1971). Following the pioneering work of Broadbent (Broadbent et al. 1961) Devine and Horton (1961) and Des Prez (Des Prez et al. 1961), the one-stage operation became more commonly known. Only after work in the 1970s and 1980s by Hodgson (1970, 1972), Asopa (Asopa et al. 1971) and Duckett (1980) did the one-stage procedure become widely accepted as routine in hypospadias surgery. The introduction by Gittes and McLaughlin in 1974 of an artificial erection test to evaluate the presence of true chordee improved the results of one-stage repairs remarkably. Preputial tissue has proved to be a valuable material for reconstruction of the neo-urethra. Following the introduction of Asopa's technique for ventral transposition of the dorsal prepuce as a pedicle flap, we undertook a study of one-stage procedures which led to the development of a technique which satisfies all the criteria for reconstruction of the several defects in hypospadias.

Patients

In the period from 1980 to 1986, 224 one-stage surgical operations for hypospadias were performed at the Royal Manchester Children's Hospital, Booth Hall Hospital and St. Mary's Hospital, Manchester, England. The 100 cases in which reconstruction was carried out using a modification of the Asopa technique are described here.

Pre-operative assessment showed the urethral meatus to be sited at the perineum in 4 patients, in the scrotum in 9, on the proximal penile shaft in 12, and at mid-shaft in 39. Distal shaft hypospadias were found in 36 patients, of whom 5 did not have chordee; varying degrees of chordee were present in all other cases. The mean age at operation was 5.0 years, the youngest patient being 1 month old and the oldest 14 years. The majority of the patients were between 3.5 and 5 years of age.

Method

The modified Asopa technique used is as follows. Under general anaesthesia, a penile block or caudal anaesthesia with bupivacaine is carried out. A 4/0 silk holding suture is passed through the glans and used subsequently to retain the 8F feeding tube which is used for urinary diversion. In some instances, holding sutures are placed on each side of the dorsal preputial hood.

The incisions for elevation of the preputial pedicle flap and mobilisation of the hypospadiac meatus are marked with Bonney's blue (Figs. 1a, b, 2, 3). Care should be taken to preserve a subcoronal preputial collar. The prepuce and the skin over the penile shaft are then extensively mobilised at the fascial plane over-

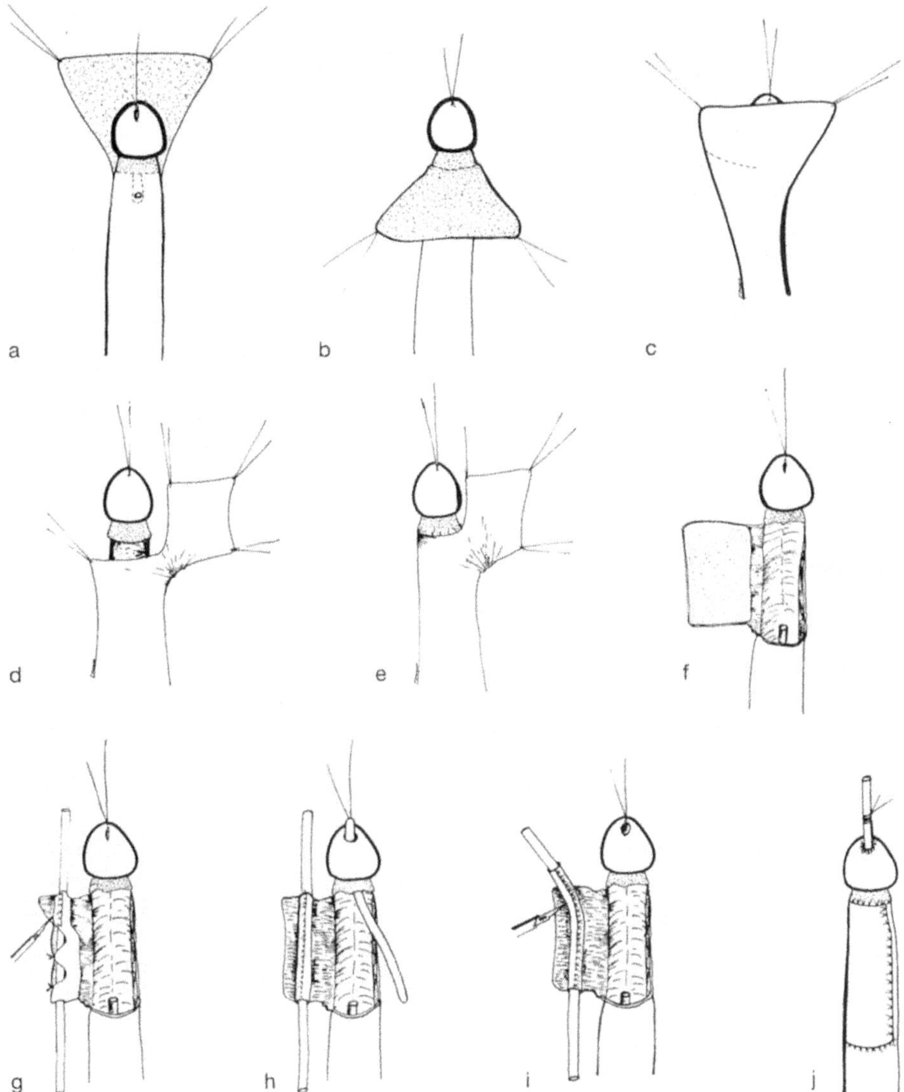

Fig. 1. a–c Proposed incisions marked with Bonney's blue. **d** Back-cut incision of the dorsal prepuce. **e** Suturing of dorsal shaft skin to the mucosal coronal cuff. **f–i** Formation of neo-urethra. **j** Completed repair

lying the corpora as far as the base of the penis (Fig. 4). The chordee is completely released, allowing the urethral meatus to migrate proximally. A 2- to 3-mm cuff of urethra is also raised. A back-cut incision is made on one side of the prepuce, extending as far as the dorsal vein (Figs. 1c, 5). Care is taken to ensure that sufficient skin is left to comfortably cover the dorsal penile shaft (Figs. 1d, 6). The pre-

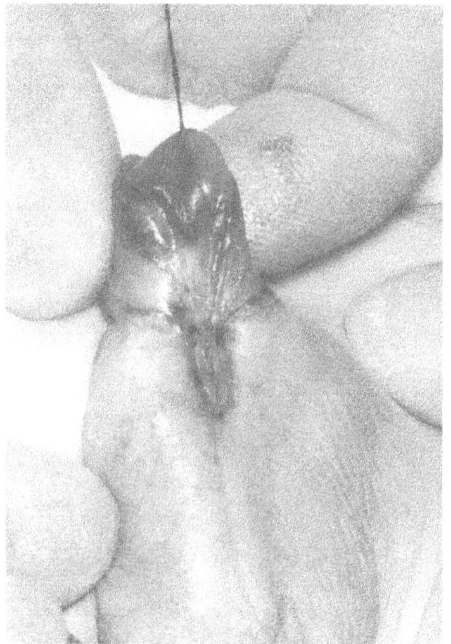

Fig. 2. Proposed incision of the ventral aspect of the penile shaft, marked with Bonney's blue

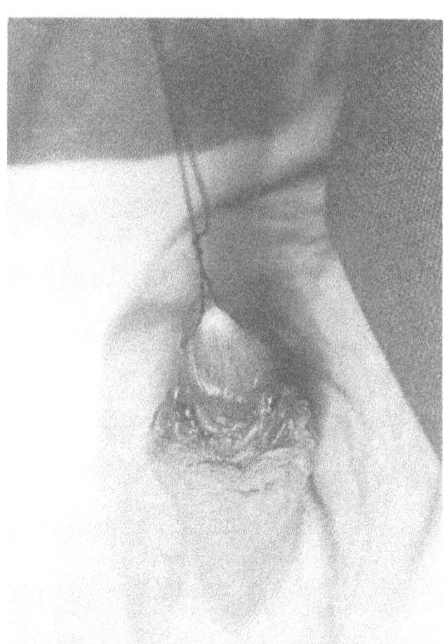

Fig. 3. Proposed incision of the dorsal aspect of the penile shaft, marked with Bonney's blue

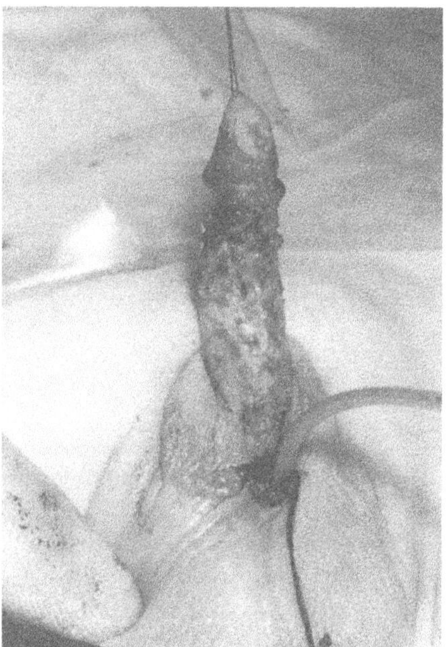

Fig. 4. Denuded penile shaft with fully mobilised prepuce

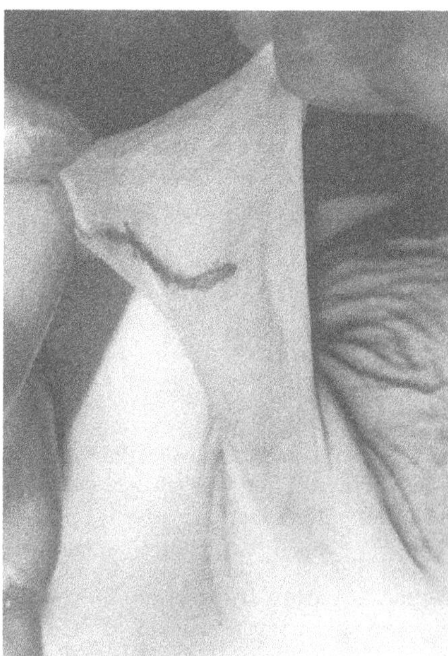

Fig. 5. Proposed back-cut incision, marked with Bonney's blue

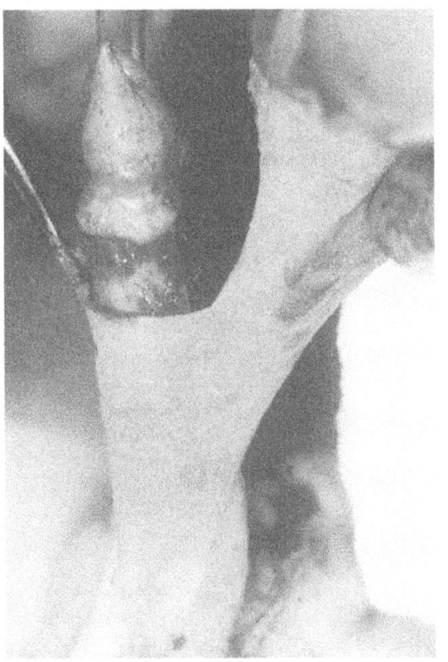

Fig. 6. Dorsal aspect after back cut

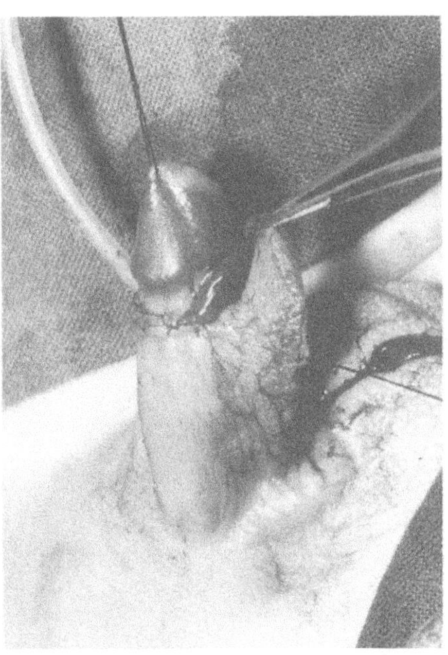

Fig. 7. Dorsal shaft skin sutured to mucosal coronal cuff

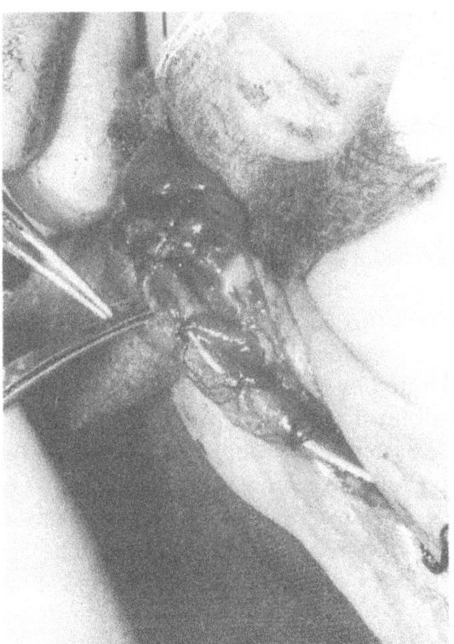

Fig. 8. Construction of neo-urethra: elevation of edges of the inner preputial layer from the outer layer

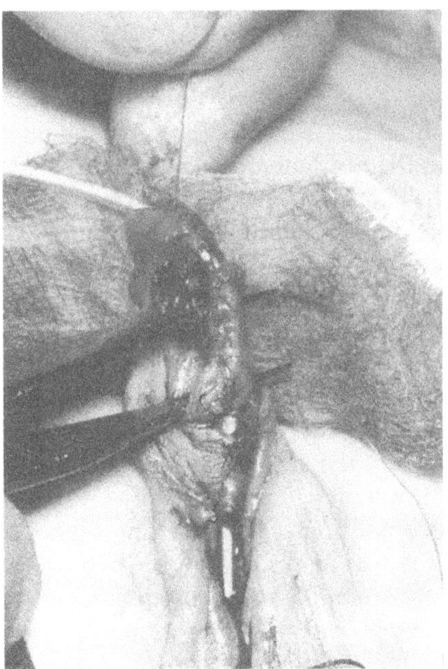

Fig. 9. Mobilisation of distal end of neo-urethra

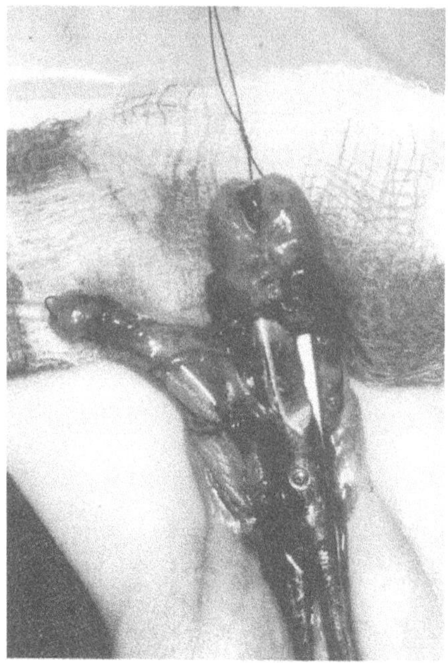

Fig. 10. Formation of sub-glandular tunnel with scissors

Fig. 11. Proximal neo-urethral–urethral anastomosis

putial flap is transposed ventrally on its pedicle and the dorsal shaft skin is sutured to the residual mucosal cuff at the corona (Figs. 1e, 7).

The inner glandular surface of the preputial flap (Fig. 1f) is incised along all its borders and the edges are elevated. A skin tube, which will become the neo-urethra, is constructed to fit comfortably around a 6F or 8F feeding tube (Figs. 1g, 8), the width depending on the child's age and the size of the penis. A continuous subcuticular or horizontal mattress inverting suture is used to ensure complete inversion of the skin edges. The distal end is mobilised (Figs. 1i, 9) and brought through a sub-glandular tunnel, which is formed by blunt dissection with a pair of scissors (Fig. 10). The dissection at corporal level extends beneath the glans, following the natural plane; the dissecting scissors are brought just beneath the meatal pit which is normally present on the glans. This pit is carefully incised at its deepest point. The resulting tunnel and meatus are graded with Hegar's dilators (Fig. 1h) to ensure that the neo-urethra will lie loosely within the tunnel. The distal portion of the neo-urethra is anastomosed to the deepest portion of the glandular meatus, carefully preserving the meatal lips. The lateral glandular elements are then brought together over the neo-urethra with two or three sutures, thus reconstructing the ventral surface of the glans. The neo-urethra is anastomosed proximally to the previously elevated urethral cuff (Fig. 11). The outer skin layer of the prepuce, still attached to the neo-urethra and sharing the same blood supply, is

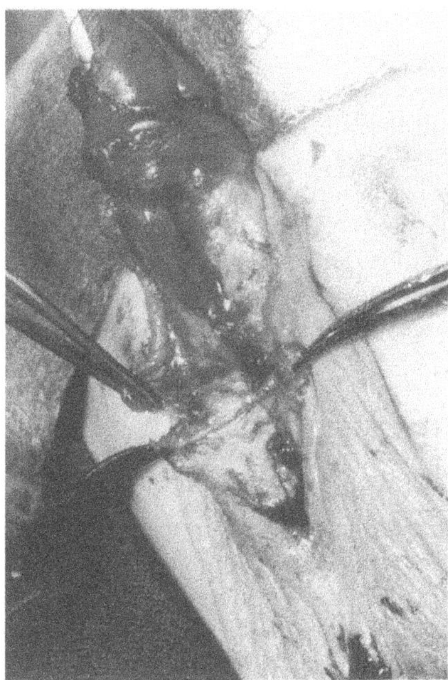

Fig. 12. Closure of ventral skin defect with outer layer of prepuce still attached to neo-urethra

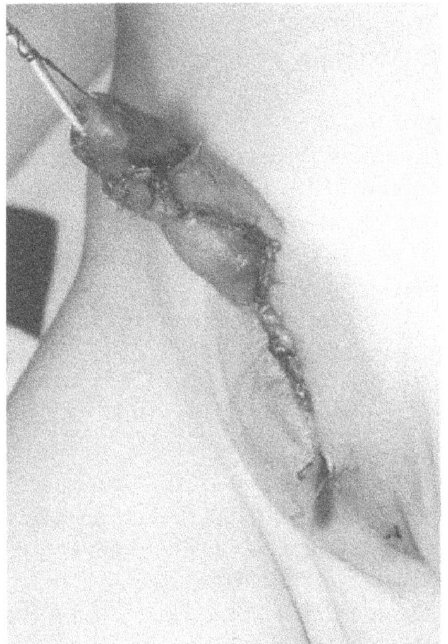

Fig. 13. Completed repair (wound drain inserted for 24 h if extensive scrotal skin mobilisation was performed)

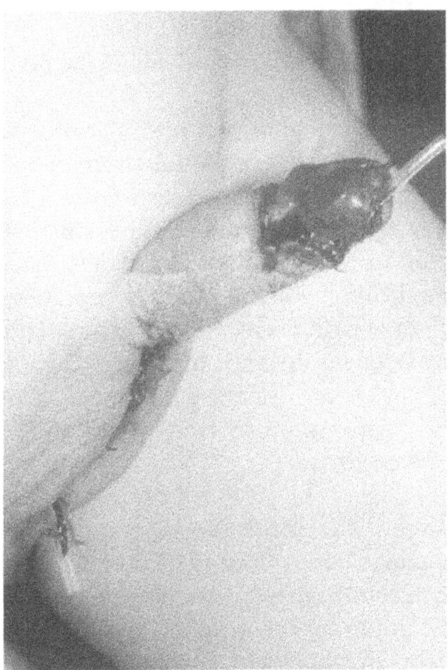

Fig. 14. 3M Micropore tape dressing (wound drain inserted for 24 h if extensive scrotal skin mobilisation was performed)

used to close the ventral penile skin defect (Fig. 1k, Fig. 12). Excessive skin is excised for better cosmetics, special care being taken not to damage the blood supply to the neo-urethra. 6/0 Dexon or 7/0 polydioxanone sutures are used throughout the whole repair.

Figure 13 illustrates the completed repair. The only dressing consists of 3M Micropore tape, running across the suture line at the ventral surface of the shaft (Fig. 14). Circumferential dressings are avoided since they may impair the blood supply. The catheter is retained until healing appears well advanced, usually for about 10 days. During this period, prophylactic antibiotics (e.g. trimethoprim and sulphametoxazone) are administered.

Results

Twenty-one patients (21%) developed fistulae. Of these, 11 had undergone repair for mid-shaft hypospadias, 8 for distal shaft hypospadias, and 2 for penoscrotal hypospadias. Six fistulae closed spontaneously; one was only minimal, at the glandular tip, and was not treated further. Ten have been repaired, while 4 are still awaiting surgery. One child developed a stricture at the neo-urethra-urethral junction, requiring further operation. Three patients developed a meatal stenosis of which one was released surgically.

Skin dehiscences occurred in two cases and these have undergone a successful second reconstruction.

In three patients torsion of the penile shaft occurred, requiring surgical correction in all cases.

No residual or recurrent chordee was seen.

The post-operative functional result − evaluating force, quality and direction of the urinary stream − was good in 77, acceptable in 10, and poor in 13 patients. Post-operative cosmetic appearance of the repair, assessed by the surgeon, was good in 55, acceptable in 31 and poor in 14. The parents felt the results of the repair to be good in 69, as acceptable in 22 and as poor in 9.

Five patients have gone through puberty, all showing full penile growth. There has been no instance of recurrent chordee in these cases.

Discussion

Despite the incidence of complications, correction of all the defects in hypospadias should be undertaken as a one-stage procedure. The technique should completely correct the chordee, reconstruct a urethral tube from tissue which has the potential for growth, and should bring the meatus to its normal site on the glans. Furthermore, it should attempt to reconstruct the glans towards normality, with special emphasis on maintaining a normal vertical meatal configuration in order to provide a concentrated urinary stream. Finally, it should import sufficient tissue to fill the often extensive ventral skin defect over the penile shaft. At the end of the procedure, having satisfied all these criteria, the appearance of the penis should be similar to that following a routine circumcision. It is obvious that correction of all defects by one operation at a young age avoids the psychological trauma (24, 17) of repeated hospitalisation and operations on a sensitive organ which have led in the past to the 'hypospadias cripple'.

The age for hypospadias repair has often been dictated by social criteria, such as school age. The majority of the patients in our series were operated on between the ages of 3.5 and 5 years. Experience with the one-stage procedure in younger age groups has led us to agreement with Belman and Kass (1982), Wacksman (1983) and Schultz et al. (1983) that operation before the end of the 1st year of life is a safe and feasible proposition. Furthermore it takes advantage of the lesser scarring and better growth potential of younger tissue. The only disadvantage of early operation relates to the smaller size of the tissues, which demands greater surgical expertise. Optical magnification (Wacksman 1984) and the pre-operative use of topical dehydrotestosterone to improve penile size and quality of tissue (Monfort and Lucas 1982; Monfort et al. 1983) have been suggested as helpful measures to reduce these difficulties.

There are points of difference between our modification of Asopa's technique and other similar repairs. Construction of the neo-urethra is performed along the transverse (occasionally oblique) axis of the pedicle flap, retaining the attachment of the inner to the outer layer of the prepuce. This causes less disruption of the vascular layer and hence ensures a much better blood supply to the neo-urethra and the skin to be used for ventral shaft cover. It has not been found necessary to island the neo-urethra as Harris (1984) and Duckett (1980) have proposed. Indeed, our clinical observation suggests that this may lead to unnecessary interference with the blood supply and, hence, the viability of the outer layer of the preputial skin.

Retention of a large part of the outer layer of preputial skin proved to be a major disadvantage, in that it led to an unnatural appearance because of excessive bulk. The technique was therefore adjusted to include resection of all excessive skin, thus giving a cosmetically acceptabe, normal-looking penile shaft. Care should be taken not to overdo this aspect of the procedure, since it may result in torsion of the penile shaft.

A most striking feature of the penis is the appearance of the glans. The hypospadiac glans is splayed ventrally and thus requires reconstruction. A more normal appearance can be achieved by rotating the lateral elements of the glans and opposing them ventrally, thus reconstructing the frenular area. Of major importance to a concentrated, 'riffled' urinary stream is a vertical meatus with well opposed meatal lips. The neo-urethra should therefore be sutured to the depth of the glandular pit, so as to preserve the well-formed meatal lips which are invariably present. This feature, combined with a neo-urethral orifice wide enough to comfortably accommodate an 8F feeding tube, has led to a marked reduction in the incidence of meatal stenosis.

We attribute the low incidence of neo-urethra—urethral strictures to the formation of a wide, tension-free anastomosis between well vascularised tissues. Inversion and accurate apposition of the anastomotic edges by subcuticular or interrupted horizontal mattress sutures are important to rapid healing and may be significant in reducing the rate of fistula formation. The fistula rate remains unacceptably high, although it compares reasonably with other authors' experiences (Kelalis 1981; Monfort et al. 1983; Ottolenghi 1984). The majority of fistulae occurred within the first group of 30 patients. Subsequent results improved as the technique and surgical skill became more established. Secondary procedures for correction of complications have proved to be relatively simple and uncomplicated, such that the vast majority of patients have required only one further intervention.

Five patients have completed puberty with no suggestion of recurrent chordee. Although this is as yet only a small number of patients and, hence, not significant, this feature is consistent with the expectation of full growth and extensibility of the vascularised full-thickness skin used for the construction of the neourethra.

In conclusion, the one-stage hypospadias repair has proved to be a major advance in hypospadias surgery. The technique, leading to a normal penile appearance, can be successfully applied to the child under 12 months of age, avoiding the psychological upset associated with repeated operative intervention on a sensitive organ in the older age groups.

References

Asopa HS, Elhence EP, Atri SP, Bansal NK (1971) One-stage correction of penile hypospadias using a foreskin tube. A preliminary report. Int Surg 55:435–440

Belman AB, Kass EJ (1982) Hypopadias repair in children less than 1 year old. J Urol 128: 1273–1274

Broadbent TR, Woolf RM, Toksu E (1961) Hypospadias: one-stage repair. Plast Reconstr Surg 27:154–159

Browne D (1953) A comparison of the Duplay and Denis Browne techniques for hypospadias operations. Surgery 34:787–798

Byars LT (1950) Surgical repair of hypospadias. Surg Clin North Am 30:1371–1378

Cecil AB (1952) Modern treatment of hypospadias. J Urol 67:1006–1011

Culp OS (1959) Experience with 200 hypospadias: evaluation of therapeutic plans. Surg Clin North Am 39:1007–1010

Des Prez JD, Persky L, Kiehn CL (1961) One stage repair of hypospadias by island flap technique. Plast Reconstr Surg 28:405–411

Devine CJ, Horton CE (1961) A one-stage hypospadias repair. J Urol 85:166–172

Duckett JW (1980) Transverse preputial island flap technique for repair of severe hypospadias. Urol Clin North Am 7:423–430

Fuqua F, Belt A (1971) Renaissance of urethroplasty: the Belt technique of hypospadias repair. J Urol 106:782–785

Gittes RF, McLaughlin AP (1974) Injection technique to induce penile erection. Urology 4: 473–474

Harris DL (1984) Splitting the prepuce to provide two independently vascularised flaps: a one-stage repair of hypospadias and congenital short urethra. Br J Plast Surg 37:108–116

Hodgson NB (1970) A one-stage hypospadias repair. J Urol 104:281–283

Hodgson NB (1972) One stage hypospadias repair surgery. Urol Proc 1:4

Kelalis PP (1981) Uréthroplastie pour hypospadias: complications des opérations en un temps ou plusieurs temps. J d'Urologie 87,2:93–96

Manley ChB, Epstein ES (1981) Early hypospadias repair. J Urol 125:698–700
Monfort G, Lucas C (1982) Dehydrotestosterone penile stimulation in hypospadias surgery. Eur Urol 8:201–203
Monfort G, Jean P, Lacoste M (1983) Correction des hypospadias postérieurs en un temps par lambeau pédicule transversal (intervention de Duckett). A propos de 50 obsérvations. Chir Pédiatr 24:71–74
Ombrédanne L (1923) Précis clinique et opératoire de chirurgie infantile, vol 1. Masson, Paris, pp 654–689
Ottolenghi A (1984) Hypospadias: considérations de tactique et de technique chirurgicales. Chir Pédiatr 25:186–188
Schultz JR, Klykylo WM, Wacksman J (1983) Timing of elective hypospadias repair in children. Pediatrics 71:342–351
Wacksman J (1983) Genital surgery timing: psychological and surgical aspects. Dialog Ped Urol 6:5
Wacksman J (1984) Results of early hypospadias surgery using optical magnification. J Urol Vol 131:516–517

Reconstruction of Foreskin
in Distal Hypospadias Repair

P. Frey[1,2] and S. J. Cohen[1]

Summary

In the period between 1980 and 1985 101 one-stage repairs for distal hypospadias
were carried out. Fifty-five patients were operated on using the Magpi technique
as originally described by Duckett (1981). The hypospadias of the remaining 46
patients were corrected using a modification of this technique incorporating reconstruction of the foreskin.

The technique of the modified, prepuce-preserving operation is described.
Despite complications such as moderate meatal stenosis, fistulae and glandular-
meatal as well as foreskin dehiscence, the overall functional and cosmetic results
were very good.

Zusammenfassung

Von 1980 bis 1985 wurden 101 distale Hypospadien in einer Sitzung operativ kor-
rigiert. 55 Patienten wurden nach der Magpi-Methode operiert, die von Duckett
(1981) beschrieben wurde. Bei den übrigen 46 Patienten kam eine Modifikation
dieser Methode mit Vorhaut-Rekonstruktion zur Anwendung.

Die Technik der modifizierten Methode zur Erhaltung der Vorhaut wird beschrieben. Trotz aufgetretener Komplikationen wie mäßiggradige Meatus-Ste-
nose, Fisteln und Glans- sowie Vorhautnaht-Dehiszenzen waren die funktionellen
und kosmetischen Ergebnisse im Ganzen sehr gut.

Résumé

Entre 1980 et 1985 nous avons pratiqué 101 interventions chirugicales en un temps
dans le but de corriger des hypospadias distales. 55 patients ont été opérés selon
la méthode Magpi, telle qu'elle a été décrite pour la première fois par Duckett
(1981). Dans le cas de 46 autres patients, cette méthode a été modifiée et com-
prend la reconstitution du prépuce.

[1]Department of Paediatric Urology, Booth Hall Children's Hospital, 9 Charlestown Road,
Blackley, Manchester M9 2AA, United Kingdom
[2]*Current address:* Kinderchirurgische Klinik, Universitäts-Kinderspital Basel, Römergasse 8,
CH-4005 Basel, Switzerland

Progress in Pediatric Surgery, Vol. 23
Ed. by L. Spitz et al.
© Springer-Verlag Berlin Heidelberg 1989

Les auteurs décrivent la méthode utilisée pour sauvegarder le prépuce. En dépit de certaines complications prévisibles, telles que sténose modérée du méat, fistules et déhiscences au niveau du gland et du méat, les résultats fonctionnels et esthétiques obtenus sont très bons.

Introduction

Distal hypospadias, in which the urethral meatus is in a glandular, coronal or sub-coronal position after release of any fibrous chordee, is by far the most common variety of hypospadias. It accounts for more than 70% of all hypospadias (Duckett 1982; Juskiewensky et al. 1983; Man et al. 1984). The typical feature of this group is the incomplete fusion of the ventral prepuce and its dorsal bunching.

Although they cause relatively minor functional disabilities, such as ventral deflection of the urinary stream and/or spraying, they do represent aesthetic and psychological problems which are often underestimated. The aim of any repair should be the reconstruction of a normal looking, adequately functioning penis, with the meatus at the tip of the glans and the prepuce reconstructed.

We therefore practise Cohen's modification of the well-established Magpi operation (meatal advancement — glanduloplasty) first described by Duckett (1981). But we always preserve and reconstruct the foreskin, providing the patient or his parents do not ask for circumcision after having had the possible operative procedures and their complications carefully explained.

Patients

Between 1980 and 1985 101 one-stage repairs for distal hypospadias were performed at the Booth Hall Children's Hospital and the Royal Manchester Children's Hospital, Manchester, England.

Most of the patients were operated on by two experienced paediatric surgeons. In 46 of the patients the hypospadias was corrected with a modified Magpi procedure and the foreskin was reconstructed. Of these, 9 presented with a glandular hypospadias, 30 with a coronal hypospadias and 7 with a sub-coronal hypospadias. The mean age at operation was 4.4 years.

The remaining 55 patients, which are not discussed in this paper, underwent the original Magpi operation.

Technique

Once general anaesthesia is established the patient is given either a penile block or caudal anaesthesia with bupivacaine. To assess the presence of chordee an erection test as described by Gittes and McLaughlin (1974) is performed. In order to minimize bleeding the ventral aspect of the glans and the ventral distal para-

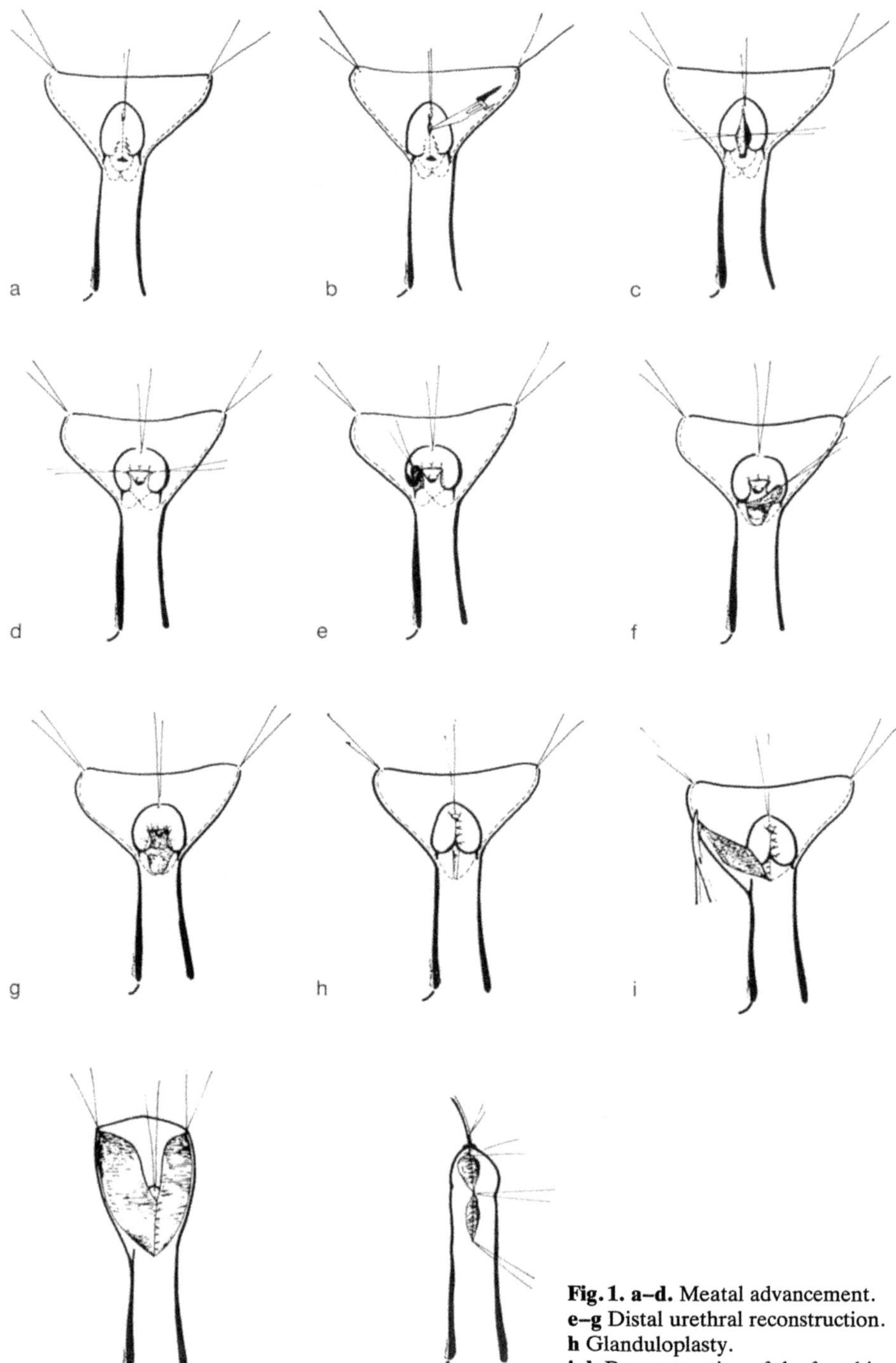

Fig. 1. a–d. Meatal advancement.
e–g Distal urethral reconstruction.
h Glanduloplasty.
i–k Reconstruction of the foreskin

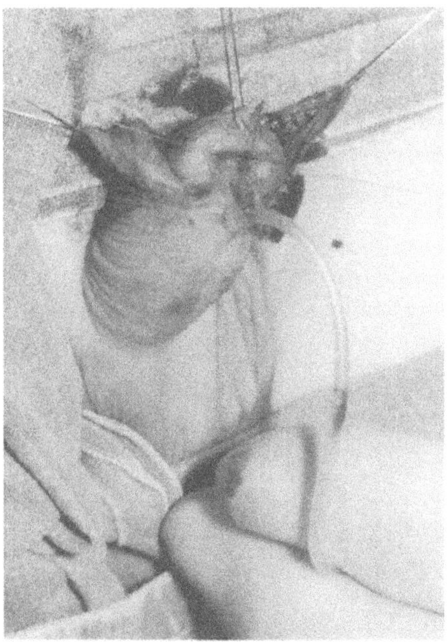

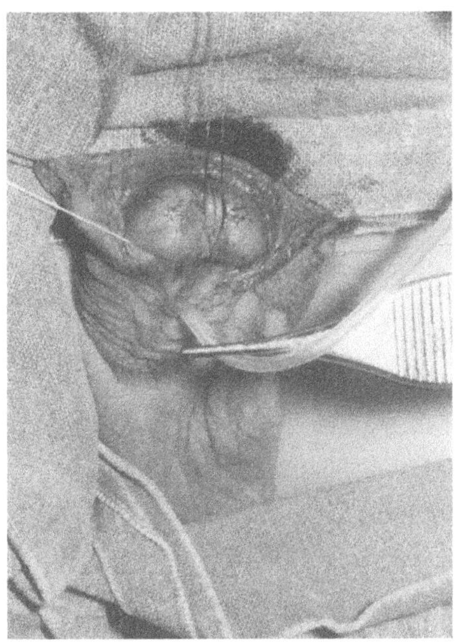

Fig. 2. Heineke-Mikulicz procedure of meatal advancement

Fig. 3. Completed meatal advancement

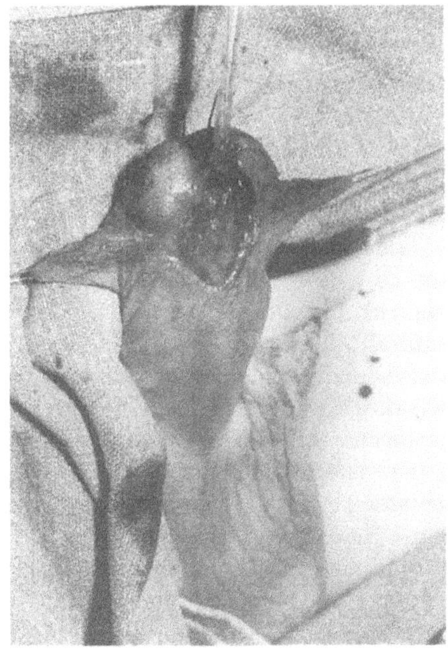

Fig. 4. Flap is raised and lifted up through 180°

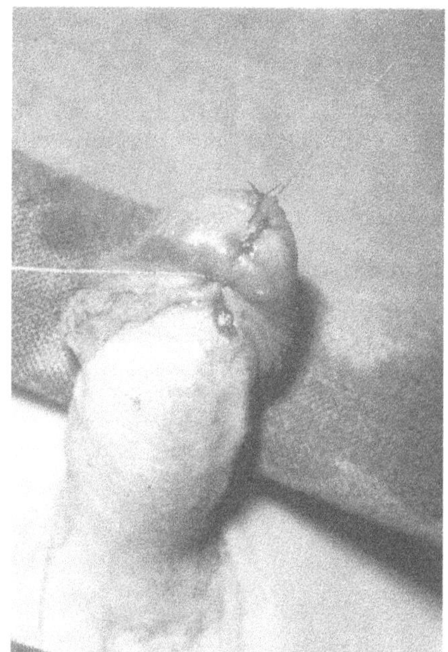

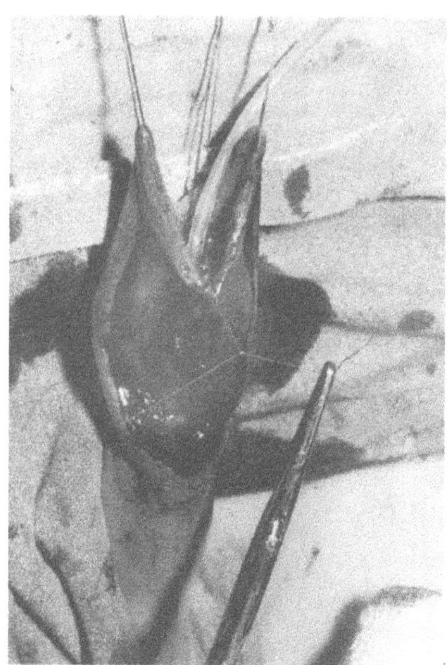

Fig. 5. Glanduloplasty completed. Notice the gaping skin defect proximal to corona which ought to be sutured before reconstruction of foreskin is carried out

Fig. 6. Sharp dissection separating the shiny mucosal layer of the prepuce from the outer skin layer

urethral tissue is infiltrated with 0.5–1 ml lignocaine 0.5% − adrenaline 1:200,000 solution.

Stay sutures using 3/0 silk are placed in the tip of the glans and in both sides of the dorsal prepucial hood, and the lines marking the planned incisions are drawn with methylene blue (Fig. 1a).

The glans is split longitudinally from the planned site of the neo-meatus, often marked by a glandular dimple, to the posterior edge of the hypospadiac meatus (Fig. 1b). Care should be taken to lay open or excise the blind-ending accessory urethral pit, occasionally found distal to the hypospadiac meatus. The gaping, longitudinally split glans is sutured transversely with polydioxanone (PDS) 6/0 or 7/0 sutures as in the Heineke-Mikulicz procedure (Figs. 1c, d, 2). Duckett's meatal advancement is now completed (Fig. 3).

The lateral glandular "ears" are well mobilised, the dissection starting from the lateral edges of the meatal advancement suture line, continuing proximally towards the corona of each side (Fig. 1e). A small flap similar to the one described by Mathieu (1932) or a flip-flap (Wacksman 1981) is raised (Figs. 1f, 4). Care is taken not to damage the urethral roof which can be extremely thin at this level. If there are fibrous bands forming chordee, these are released. The raised flap is

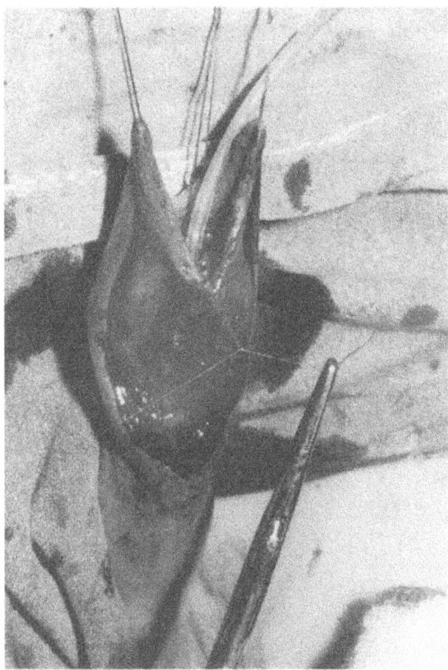

Fig. 7. Reconstruction of inner mucosal layer of prepuce

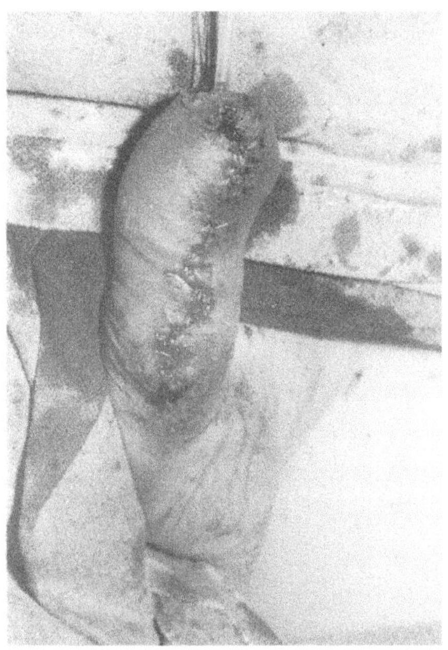

Fig. 8. Completed repair: outer aspect of foreskin

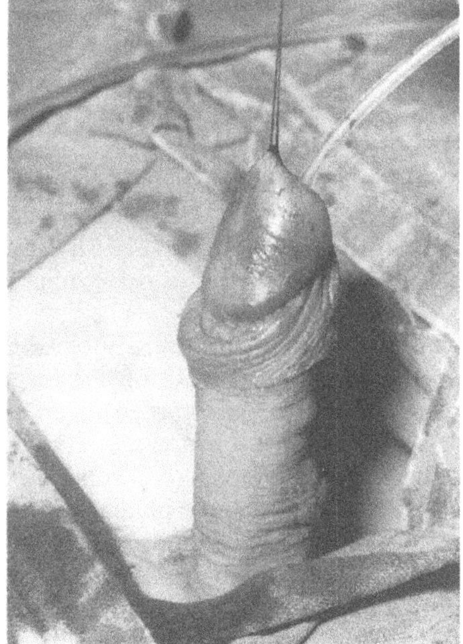

Fig. 9. Completed repair: retracted foreskin

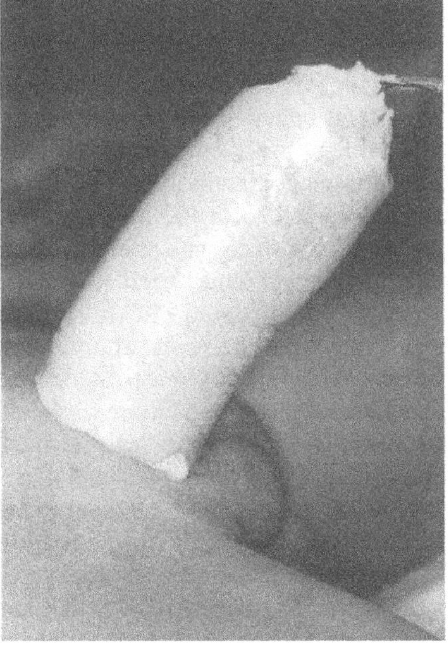

Fig. 10. Silastic foam dressing applied

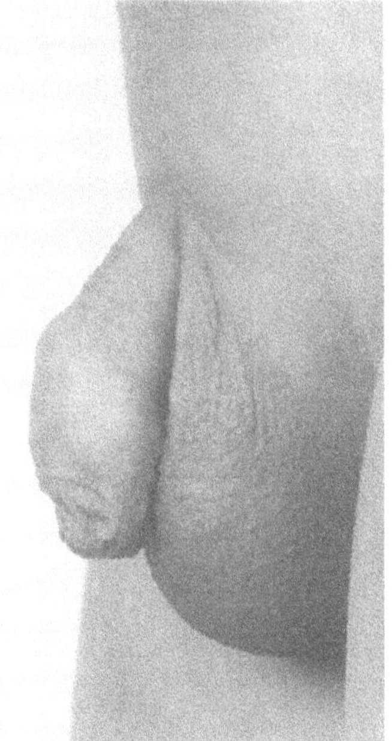

Fig. 11. Repair 2 months post-operatively: outer aspect

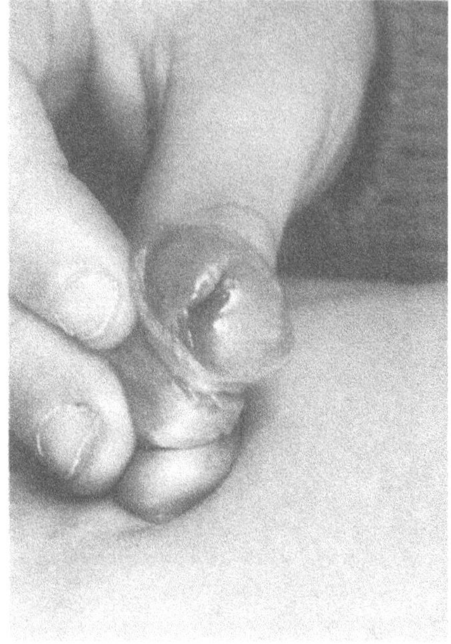

Fig. 12. Repair 2 months post-operatively: glandular aspect with retracted foreskin

fixed with two PDS 7/0 sutures to the under surface of the mobilised glans at the two lateral edges of the meatal advancement suture line. Single sutures then fix either side of the lateral edges of the flap to the penile fascia, having been exposed following glandular mobilisation (Fig. 1g). The mobilised glans is adapted over the neo-urethra with PDS 6/0 sutures, starting at the corona. The distal ventral neo-urethra is fixed with the most distal suture of the glans repair (Fig. 1h). The glanduloplasty is completed (Fig. 5). The skin defect proximal to the corona is closed with interrupted PDS 6/0 sutures.

At this point the inner, shiny mucosal layer of the foreskin is separated from the outer skin layer by sharp dissection with pointed scissors (Fig. 1i, 6). The inner layer is mobilised and approximated with continuous or interrupted inverting sutures (Fig. 1j, 7). After careful haemostasis the outer layer of the foreskin is closed (Fig. 1k). Figures 8 and 9 illustrate the completed repair. A feeding tube (e.g. no. 6) can be left in the bladder and is fixed with the glandular holding suture. As a dressing we prefer silastic foam (Fig. 10) or 3M Micropore applied directly to the wound. If the latter is used care should be taken only to dress the hemicircumference, to prevent venous and lymphatic congestion.

Figures 11 and 12 illustrate the result of the repair two months post-operatively.

Results

The post-operative follow-up of the 46 patients who underwent hypospadias repair and reconstruction of the prepuce showed the following complications:

Five patients developed a minor fistula. One of these closed spontaneously; another was very close to the neo-meatus and did not require repair.

Mild stenosis of the neo-meatus was present in another five cases but resolved after one or two urethral dilatations.

Meatal-glandular dehiscences were seen in six boys; three of them were only of cosmetic relevance.

Of the 10 cases where dehiscence of the foreskin occurred, one required circumcision and six needed further repair. The remaining three showed only minimal dehiscence at the tip.

Wound infection with *Escherichia coli* developed once. We therefore treated all our hypospadias repairs prophylactically for 5 days with trimethoprim and sulphametoxazole. None of the patients developed a secondary phimosis.

Twelve patients required a second operation, three of them due to functional, nine due to cosmetic reasons. A third operation was necessary in one case in which a fistula reoccurred.

The overall functional result — evaluating the force, quality and direction of the urinary stream — was very good or good in 89.1% of cases and acceptable in 10.9%. There were no poor functional results. The cosmetic-aesthetic appearance of the reconstructed penis, as assessed by the surgeon, was very good or good in 73.9% of cases, acceptable in 15.2% and poor in 10.9%. The patient or his parents judged the post-operative result of the repair as very good or good in 78.3%, acceptable in 15.2% and poor 6.5%.

Discussion

Out of a variety of operative techniques which have been described for distal hypospadias repair — procedures involving either constructing a new skin tube (Kim and Hendren 1981; King 1970, 1981; Mustardé 1965) or raising a ventral proximal skin flap (Mathieu 1932; Ombrédanne 1932; Konrad and Neisius 1985) — we prefer Duckett's Magpi procedure if circumcision is requested and for all cases without fibrous chordee or "skin chordee."

However, the goal of our repair is the reconstruction of a normal penis: normal in appearance and in function, as demanded by Duckett and many other authors. But in addition we try to reconstruct a normal-looking foreskin. We therefore perform the technique described above in all cases in which we pre-operatively decide for the reconstruction of the foreskin as well as when we intra-operatively find fibrous chordee or "skin chordee" requiring release.

Agreeing with Maier's findings (W. A. Maier, 1986, personal communication), we found in our series a surprisingly high demand for preservation of the foreskin after we had explained to the patient and parents the possibility of preputial reconstruction. Maybe, the Old World is more conscious than the New of the beauty of a well-reconstructed, normal-looking foreskin!

We are fully aware that in our series the complication rate is higher than what is normally stated in the literature. We believe that this is due to the fact that our complications, evaluated by very careful and self-critical post-operative assessment, also include very minor complications as well as these which arose during the learning period. All the same, the closure of a fistula, the repair of a dehiscence or the dilatation of a meatal stenosis are only minor procedures and can be done as day surgery cases. Almost 100% of our cases overall proved to be functionally and cosmetically successful after the occasionally necessary secondary minor procedure.

Agreeing with Schultz et al. (1983) and Wacksman (1984) in their evaluation of the psychological trauma caused by the operation, and on the basis of our own findings regarding functional and cosmetic results, we believe that distal hypospadias repair should be performed either in early infancy, between 9 and 15 months, or between the ages of 2.5 and 3 years. The very early operation certainly requires the use of magnifying loops or operating microscopes, which as yet is not common practice.

References

Duckett JW (1981) Magpi (Meatal advancement and glanuloplasty). A procedure for sub-coronal hypospadias. Urol Clin North Am 8:513–520

Duckett JW (1982) Current trends in urology, vol 2. Williams and Wilkins, Baltimore, pp 16–30

Gittes RF, McLaughlin AP (1974) Injection technique to introduce penile erection. Urology 4: 473–475

Juskiewensky S, Vaysse Ph, Guitard J, Moscovi J (1983) Traitment des hypospadias antérieurs. Chir Pédiatr 24:75–79

Kim SH, Hendren WH (1981) Repair of mild hypospadias. J Pediatr Surg 16(6):806–811

King LR (1970) Hypospadias – a one stage repair without skin graft based on a new principle: chordee is sometimes produced by skin alone. J Urol 103:660–662

King LR (1981) Cutaneous chordee and its implications in hypospadias repair. Urol Clin North Am 8:397–402

Konrad G, Neisius D (1985) Mikrochirurgische Hypospadiekorrektur im Säuglings- und Kleinkindalter. Ethicon GmbH, Norderstedt, FRG, pp 3–23 (Im Dienste der Chirurgie, no. 48)

Man DWK, Hamdy MH, Bissett WH (1984) Experience with meatal advancement and glanuloplasty (Magpi) hypospadias repair. Br J Urol 56:70–72

Mathieu P (1932) Traitment en un temps de l'hypospadias balanique et juxta-balanique. J Chir 39:481–484

Mustardé JC (1965) One stage correction of distal hypospadias and other peoples fistulae. Br J Plast Surg 18:413–422

Ombrédanne L (1932) Précis clinique et opératoire de chirurgie infantile. Masson, Paris, pp 817–836

Schultz JR, Klykylo WM, Wacksman J (1983) Timing of elective hypospadias repair in children. Pediatrics 71:342–351

Wacksman J (1981) Modification of the one stage flip-flap procedure to repair distal penile hypospadias. Urol Clin North Am 8:527–530

Wacksman J (1984) Results of early hypospadias surgery using optical magnifications. J Urol 131:516–517

Progress in Pediatric Surgery

Volume 21

P. Wurnig (Ed.)

Trachea and Lung Surgery in Childhood

1987. 75 figures. X, 147 pages. ISBN 3-540-17232-7

Contents: *B. Minnigerode, H. G. Richter:* Pathophysiology of Subglottic Tracheal Stenosis in Childhood. – *M. Marcovich, F. Pollauf, K. Burian:* Subglottic Stenosis in Newborns After Mechanical Ventilation. – *R. N. P. Berkovits, E. J. van der Schans, J. C. Molenaar:* Treatment of Congenital Cricoid Stenosis. – *E. Hof:* Surgical Correction of Laryngotracheal Stenoses in Children. – *R. N. P. Berkovits, N. M. A. Bax, E. J. van der Schans:* Surgical Treatment of Congenital Laryngotracheo-oesophageal Cleft. – *S. E. Haugen, T. Kufaas, S. Svenningsen:* Free Periosteal Grafts in Tracheal Reconstruction: An Experimental Study. – *R. Daum, H. J. Denecke, H. Roth:* Tumour-Induced Intraluminal Stenoses of the Cervical Trachea – Tumour Excision and Tracheoplasty. – *I. Louhimo, M. Leijala:* Cardiopulmonary Bypass in Tracheal Surgery in Infants and Small Children. – *T. A. Angerpointner, W. Stelter, K. Mantel, W. Ch. Hecker:* Resection of an Intrathoracic Tracheal Stenosis in a Child. – *G. M. Salzer, H. Hartl, P. Wurnig:* Treatment of Tracheal Stenoses by Resection in Infancy and Early Childhood. – *H. Halsband:* Long-Distance Resection of the Trachea with Primary Anastomosis in Small Children. – *K. Gdanietz, K. Vorpahl, G. Piehl, A. Höck:* Clinical Symptoms and Treatment of Lung Separation. – *M. Leijala, I. Louhimo:* Extralobar Sequestration of the Lung in Children. – *E. Horcher, F. Helmer:* Scimitar Syndrome and Associated Pulmonary Sequestration: Report of a Successfully Corrected Case. – *M. R. Becker, F. Schindera, W. A. Maier:* Congenital Cystic Adenmatoid Malformation of the Lung. – *W. Tischer, H. Reddemann, P. Herzog, K. Gdanietz, J. Witt, P. Wurnig, A. Reiner:* Experience in Surgical Treatment of Pulmonary and Bronchial Tumours in Childhood. – *N. Augustin, S. Hofmann-v. Kap-Herr, P. Wurnig:* Endotracheal and Endobronchial Tumours in Childhood.

This volume deals with the new and special challenges posed by trachea surgery in children. The recent improvements in respiratory therapy and intensive care have facilitated observation of congenital malformations and various acquired pathological deformities of the trachea and bronchi. The contributions presented here report on these important observations and discuss the problems involved, together with possible solutions. Cases of surgical pulmonary diseases are also reviewed (except for the already widely discussed problems of empyemas and bronchiectasis).

Springer-Verlag
Berlin Heidelberg New York
London Paris Tokyo Hong Kong

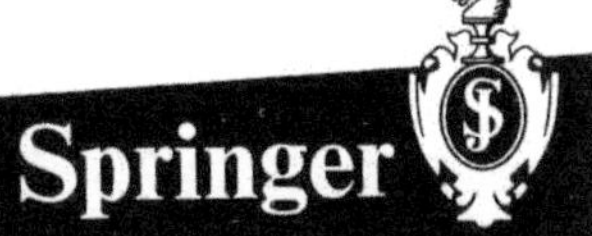

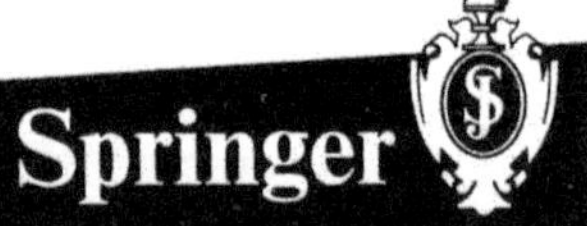

Springer

GPSR Compliance
The European Union's (EU) General Product Safety Regulation (GPSR) is a set
of rules that requires consumer products to be safe and our obligations to
ensure this.

If you have any concerns about our products, you can contact us on

ProductSafety@springernature.com

In case Publisher is established outside the EU, the EU authorized
representative is:

Springer Nature Customer Service Center GmbH
Europaplatz 3
69115 Heidelberg, Germany